NO LAUGHING MATTER
HISTORICAL ASPECTS OF ANAESTHESIA

NO LAUGHING MATTER
HISTORICAL ASPECTS OF ANAESTHESIA

Catalogue of an exhibition
held at
the Wellcome Institute for the History of Medicine
8 June to 25 September 1987

By

Christopher Lawrence and Ghislaine Lawrence

with the assistance of

Huw Geddes and
Lorraine Ward

Wellcome Institute for the History of Medicine/Science Museum

London
1987

ISBN 0 85484 056 7

CONTENTS

Acknowledgements .... p. 7
A Note on the Catalogue Entries and Abbreviations .... p. 9
Introduction .... p. 11
Images of Anaesthesia: Priority (Case 1) .... p. 14
Images of Anaesthesia: Precursors (Case 2) .... p. 16
Images of Anaesthesia: Celebrations (Case 3) .... p. 19
Images of Anaesthesia: Public Perceptions (Case 4) .... p. 22
Anaesthesia and the Victorians (Case 5) .... p. 24
Anaesthesia and Innovation (Case 6) .... p. 30
Anaesthesia and Technical Solutions (Case 7) .... p. 36
Anaesthesia and Women (Case 8) .... p. 41
Anaesthesia and Two World Wars (Case 9) .... p. 47
Anaesthesia and a New Century (Case 10) .... p. 52
Anaesthesia and Industry: One (Case 11) .... p. 56
Anaesthesia and Industry: Two (Case 12) .... p. 60
Anaesthesia and the Chloroform Question (Case 13) .... p. 63
Anaesthesia and the Cardiologist (Case 14) .... p. 67
Monitoring in Anaesthesia (Case 15) .... p. 69
Free-Standing Objects .... p. 73
Bibliography .... p. 75

ACKNOWLEDGEMENTS

An exhibition on the history of anaesthesia was first suggested to us by the the British organizers of the Second International Symposium on the History of Anaesthesia, held at the Royal College of Surgeons of England, in July 1987. The final result of that suggestion brought together artefacts from a variety of sources and assistance from a number of people. We thank all those who lent artefacts and they are acknowledged in the appropriate entries. To the Wellcome Museum of the History of Medicine at the Science Museum we owe many thanks, in particular to Lorraine Ward and Andrew Mackay, and for last minute assistance to Heather Mayfield and Timothy Boon. The exhibition at the Wellcome Institute was designed and mounted by Huw Geddes, who also designed the catalogue. His skills have been invaluable. From the Iconographic Collections at the Institute, William Schupbach and Trudy Prescott have been of great help as, of course, has the photographer, Chris Carter. For his organizational assistance we should like to thank Robin Price, Deputy Librarian. To the bibliographical knowledge and proof-reading skills of John Symons we are indebted. We should also like to record all the kindness and assistance rendered to us by Richard Ellis and David Wilkinson, from the Department of Anaesthetics at St. Bartholomew's Hospital. Finally, but not least, thanks to Marika Antoniw for sitting patiently at the word processor.

Christopher Lawrence
Wellcome Institute for
the History of
Medicine

Ghislaine Lawrence
Wellcome Museum of the
History of Medicine at
the Science Museum

1987

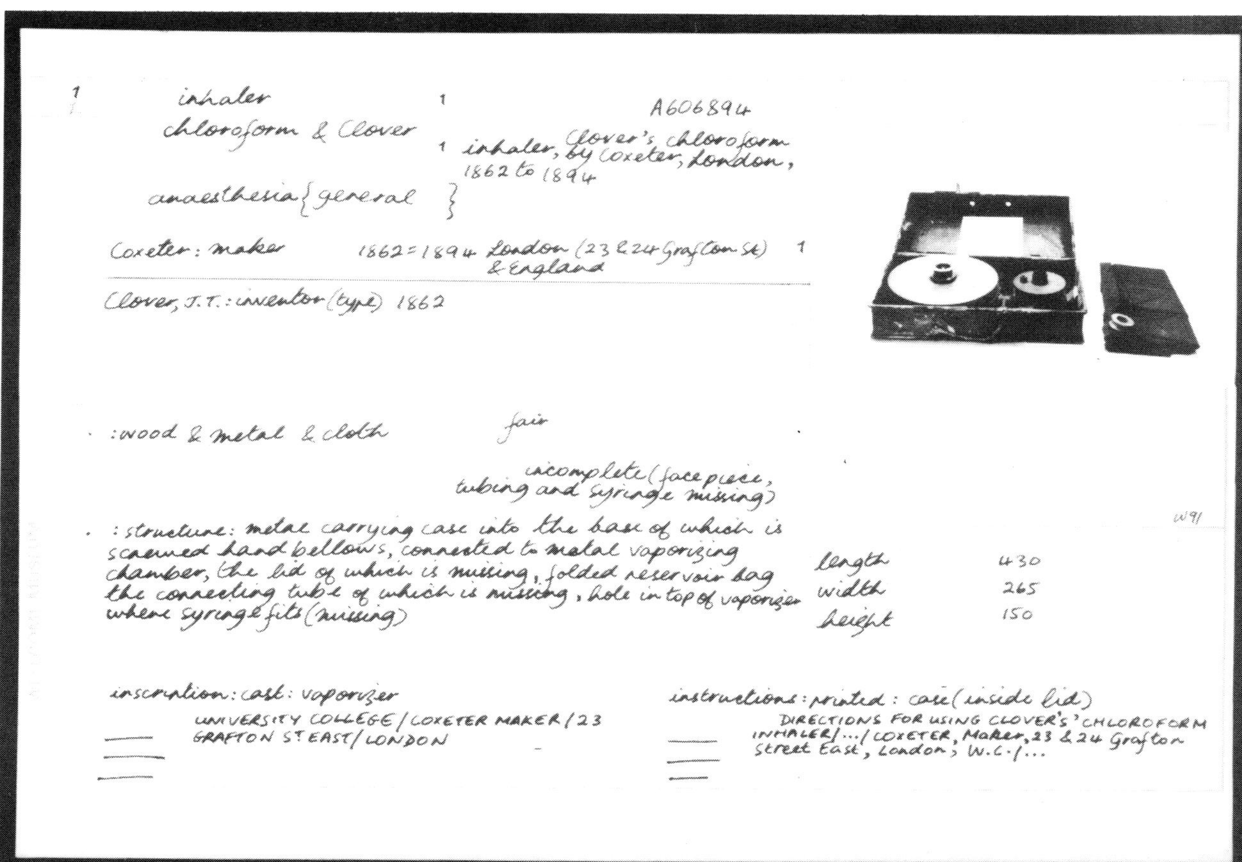

Catalogue Card

Computer Print-Out

```
A651850: Anaesthetic inhaler, for use with ether or choloroform, probably
   English, 1850-1900
   SUBJECT     : anaesthesia (general)
   SIMPLE NAME: inhalers
   INDEX TERMS: ether; chloroform
   PRODUCTION : England, 1850      -1900
   ASSOCIATION: Bailey, Dr. Henry James. - Hants: Bishopstoke, 1870      -1933
          (approx.). - owner, died 1933
   CONDITION  : good: complete
   MATERIAL   : frame: zinc; padding: cloth; case: rubber


A652176 Pt  17: Box containing five ampoules of morphine, two broken, from
   garrison at Grandenz, German, 1910-1915
   SUBJECT     : military (general medicine)
   SIMPLE NAME: anaesthetic injection ampoules
   INDEX TERMS: morphine
   PRODUCTION : Germany, 1910      -1915
   MATERIAL   : box: cardboard; ampoules: glass
   INSCR.(1)  : label - printed - lid
      Festungslazarett Graudenz/10 zugeschmol[.]zene Glasrohrenzn/0.02g
      Morphinum/hydrochloricum/in losung von 1ccm., keinfrei gemacht/1915


A652176 Pt  18: Box contain ten ampoules of morphine, three broken, from No.1
   Army Corps, German, 1910-1918
   SUBJECT     : military (general medicine)
   SIMPLE NAME: anaesthetic injection ampoules
   INDEX TERMS: morphine
   PRODUCTION : Germany, 1910      -1918
   MATERIAL   : box: cardboard: ampoules: glass
```

See opposite for a description

A NOTE ON THE CATALOGUE ENTRIES AND ABBREVIATIONS

Almost all of the books and the two-dimensional material in the exhibition come from the Library of the Wellcome Institute for the History of Medicine. Most of the museum objects come from the Wellcome Museum of the History of Medicine at the Science Museum. Both Library and Museum are based on the historical medical collections amassed by Sir Henry Wellcome (1853–1936) in the early decades of this century, together with additions made after 1936. Since 1976 the museum objects have been deposited on permanent loan to the Science Museum by the Wellcome Trustees. Museum items in the Wellcome collections prior to 1976 are distinguished by inventory numbers prefixed 'A'. Since 1976, the Science Museum has collected in its own right in the field of medical history and objects added to the collections after that date bear inventory numbers prefixed by the year of acquisition.

A significant addition to the Science Museum's collections was made in 1983, when the Royal College of Surgeons of England deposited most of their post-Listerian holdings, together with some others, on permanent loan. These all bear the inventory number – 1983/881, a further number distinguishing individual items. The Royal College of Surgeons loan included anaesthetic items largely derived from two sources (Thompson, 1962: 269). Over seventy pieces, comprising the collection of Dr. D.W. Buxton (1855–1931) were presented to the College by his son in 1932. A further twelve items came from Dr. R.J. Probyn-Williams (1866–1952) in 1936–7.

All objects owned, or held on permanent loan, by the Wellcome Museum at the Science Museum are included in the catalogue of their holdings, prepared between 1977 and 1986 and stored on computer. The catalogue contains detailed physical descriptions of the objects, together with all available further information, and the entries are exhaustive in a way that those in this Catalogue cannot be. Further enquiries regarding the objects displayed may be directed to the Wellcome Museum at the Science Museum, quoting the inventory number. An example of the catalogue cards used there, and of one format for computer print-out, are shown in the photographs on the opposite page.

Unless otherwise stated, all the books, manuscripts and pictures (of any sort) described and shown here are from the Wellcome Institute Library. Other owners of original photographs are indicated. Dates for individuals in the catalogue are given at their first mention in any new section. Makers' names, when italicized, are in the form in which they appear on the object concerned.

ABBREVIATIONS

Institutions:

RSM	Royal Society of Medicine.
WFA	Wellcome Foundation Archives.
WHL	Wellcome Institute for the History of Medicine Library.
WHMM	Wellcome Historical Medical Museum.
WIA	Wellcome Institute Archives.
WLMS	Wellcome Institute Library, Western Manuscript Collection.
WMSM	Wellcome Museum for the History of Medicine at the Science Museum.

Journals:

BJA	British Journal of Anaesthesia
BMJ	The British Medical Journal
Pharm. J.	Pharmaceutical Journal

INTRODUCTION

Among medical specialists, anaesthetists might justly claim to have taken the greatest interest in the history of their own discipline. Physicians and surgeons, of course, have produced a distinguished roll of historical authors: William Osler, Clifford Allbutt, Zachary Cope and many others. Considered in proportion to its size and recent origin however, anaesthetics is an historical industry. In Britain and America anaesthetists have formed historical societies and there is sufficient global interest in the subject to support a regular international symposium, the first of which attracted over 120 papers (Rupreht, 1985).

It is scarcely surprising that anaesthetists become interested in history in the course of their work. In no other specialty, perhaps, are practitioners so often reminded of their past. Until recently almost every standard anaesthetic text or monograph began with an historical synopsis. Moreover, the daily activity of anaesthetists surrounds them with dozens of pieces of eponymous apparatus. With a couple of exceptions, practically every object described by Bryn Thomas in the Charles King collection of historical anaesthetic apparatus is named after its inventor, almost always a practising anaesthetist (Thomas, 1975).

The interest shown by anaesthetists in the history of their subject is not recent, indeed it began at the very time that inhalational anaesthesia began to be employed on any scale. No sooner had Horace Wells (1815–48) used nitrous oxide at the Massachusetts General Hospital in 1845, and William Morton (1819–68) demonstrated ether at the same place in 1846, than a host of other characters appeared, claiming their share of credit for the discovery. The result was a vigorous and vicious pamphlet war, which went over and over, in great detail, the use of inhalational anaesthesia in the mid-1840s (Fulton, 1946). To the protagonists, this tug-of-war was not simply a question of historical punctiliousness; the outcome meant the difference between worldly success or failure, immortality or obscurity. Nor did the controversy end with the deaths of the major participants. Subsequent generations of anaesthetists have continued to debate such questions as whether Wells was hard done by, or whether Charles Jackson (1805–80) (who claimed he had told Morton about ether) was a rogue. In addition to surveying this ground, more recent historical activity has uncovered many new claimants and precursors – Crawford Long (1815–78) and Henry Hill Hickman (1800–30) for example. It has also discovered new instances of injustice, such as the neglect of David Waldie's (1813–89) part in James Young Simpson's (1811–70) discovery of chloroform anaesthesia in 1847, and the underestimated role of Gardner Quincy Colton (1814–98) and Thomas Wiltberger Evans (1823–97) in reintroducing nitrous oxide as an anaesthetic agent in the 1860s.

At least one of the reasons for this perennial interest in the history of invention, discovery, and priority in anaesthesia lies in the wider history of medicine. In the nineteenth century, doctors developed and used two quite different accounts of their work. In one of these, science and medicine were described as international, collaborative and anonymous enterprises devoted to the accumulation of knowledge for the service of humanity. In the other, these pursuits were seen as theatres of heroism in which great individuals, by dint of genius or courage, made huge leaps forward in the understanding of disease or in the practical relief of suffering or, even better, in both. To the Victorians, individualism and competition were as necessary to science and medicine as they were to commerce and industry.

Modern surgery, especially American surgery, and inhalational anaesthesia were created within this context. By the end of the nineteenth century the use of anaesthesia and asepsis permitted long, and frequently successful, operations within the body cavities. Surgery, from being a slightly inferior form of medical practice, became a powerful and prestigious occupation. Surgeons often appraised the history of their discipline, including the discovery of anaesthesia, by using the heroic account. For instance, Frederic Dennis (1850–1934), Professor of Clinical Surgery at Cornell University, wrote in 1905:

Among the important events in the history of mankind which have been far-reaching and beneficent in their influence, the discovery of anesthesia easily stands in the foremost ranks. What greater blessing has science ever conferred upon the human race? Other discoveries and inventions have indeed been revolutionary in their results for social advancement and comfort; but anesthesia outranks them all, in its combinations of kindness and power at a point of unutterable need (Dennis, 1905: 8).

Given that this was a widely shared appraisal, it is hardly surprising that much ink was spilled over what another author called "the greatest discovery of the age". Indeed the same author went on to wonder, "who is entitled to the credit of it?" (Smith, 1859). So important was the discovery of anaesthesia perceived to be, that it provoked national as well as individual claims. Dennis and many others saw anaesthesia as the product of a unique, American spirit:

This wonderful boon to suffering humanity, now grateful in use throughout the civilized world, comes from our own land – America. No other nation has presumed to lay the slightest claim to any priority in its dicovery. Anesthesia with its worldwide blessings is confessedly American (Dennis, 1905: 8).

Although most current histories of anaesthesia have abandoned this sort of heroic and chauvinistic rhetoric, concern with priority, and with individual and national contributions are still central to a great deal of contemporary scholarship. In careful hands, this has produced some very fine detective work into the lives of nineteenth century doctors (for example Cartwright, 1952; Sykes, 1960, 1961, 1982; Smith, 1982). It has also been the basis of two excellent studies of anaesthetic apparatus (Duncum, 1947; Thomas, 1975).

Paradoxically, what the best work in this genre has shown is that the scrupulous researcher ends up discovering, not who discovered anaesthesia, but the truth of the cliché that history is a seamless web. Fine-textured study reveals that, in order to give a satisfactory account of the history of anaesthesia, innumerable people seem to require acknowledgment, and endless aspects of the historical process seem to need description. It turns out to be no more possible to say who discovered inhalational anaesthesia, and where and when, than it is to find a moment when oxygen was discovered or cells first described (Schaffer, 1985; Jacyna, 1983). Indeed it is likely that a sound piece of historical research could be pursued on the theory that anaesthesia was not widely perceived as very significant in the late 1840s and only in the 1850s was its discovery designated as a momentous event. In other words, heroes, discoverers and discoveries, are not things that historians *find* in the past, but things they *make*, by selection. This process of selection, now, as much as in the nineteenth century, is often ordered by such things as implicit evaluations of modern medicine, nationalism, and tacit acceptance of current models of how science works. Accounts of medicine and anaesthesia in the past, therefore, can all too easily become ways of endorsing contemporary values and current practice.

Although the discovery and invention approach to the history of anaesthesia has produced some excellent studies, it has also had less satisfactory consequences. For one thing, it has largely kept attention focused on the high spots, for instance anaesthetics given to famous men or operations performed by distinguished surgeons. A similar difficulty has also attended the study of anaesthetic objects. The preoccupation with eminence, although generating a healthy preserving interest, has sometimes led to a sort of instrument fetishism. It has become important to see, touch or, even better, possess, Augustus Waller's (1856–1922) original chloroform balance or the actual apparatus used when Edward VII had his appendix out. Previous exhibitions on the history of anaesthesia, of which there seem to have been many, have customarily adopted these approaches.

Sadly, much of the humdrum world of historical anaesthesia remains a vast, undiscovered country, a failing which can be laid at the door of anaesthetists and professional historians alike. We still know next to nothing of day-to-day anaesthetic practice in the past, who the anaesthetists were, what they used, who their suppliers were and how much anaesthetic agents cost. We know equally little about anaesthesia and the medical curriculum, professionalization, the effects of war and, until very recently, the context of the debate on the use of anaesthetics in childbirth. The latter has usually been painted in two colours only: those of religious bigotry and scientific humanism (cf. Youngson, 1979, and Pernick, 1985). An exhibition is not a good place to start thinking differently about some of these things. By their very nature exhibitions are highly selective, and most of the objects which are preserved are those with distinguished associations. Besides, it seems probable that, in many countries until well into the twentieth century, most anaesthetics were given on a cloth or a handkerchief, and an exhibition of machines must, necessarily, be distorting. In addition, as all museum curators know, but few admit in catalogues, objects are often chosen because they are sculpturally attractive, or rejected because they do not fit in the display case.

All these things notwithstanding, we have tried to organize a slightly different exhibition on anaesthesia in history. Instead of mounting a chronicle, identifying invention and discovery, we have tried to look tangentially at some of the relations of anaesthesia; for instance to surgery, to war, to women and to industry. Similarly, in the place where the visitor might expect the familiar catalogue of heroes, we have attempted to do something different and look at how the heroes have been made and displayed in texts, pictures and previous exhibitions. We have also tried to give a hint of another whole domain that begs investigation: public perceptions of anaesthesia and anaesthetists. In *Anaesthesia and the Cardiologists, Monitoring*, and *the Chloroform Question* we have perhaps been more traditional. Even here, though, we hope we have stimulated some thoughts about the history of such things as record keeping and standardization. By the very nature of the material available to us, the focus of the exhibition has been Great Britain. We have, however, attempted wherever possible to refer to the world stage. We have also tried to give some critical evaluation of the literature we have used, of which there is a bibliography.

Finally, we hope we have produced a volume that, although useful as a conventional catalogue, employs some of the less assertive, more questioning approaches which might be more appropriate to under-researched subjects. In doing this we have tried to break down some of the categories that govern and divide the literary products generated by museums and those produced by traditional historians. Definitive is the last word we would use about this volume, indeed we hope that some of its very indecisiveness will be the spur to anaesthetists and historians alike to explore those areas in the history of anaesthesia which have been so often neglected.

CASE 1:   IMAGES OF ANAESTHESIA: PRIORITY

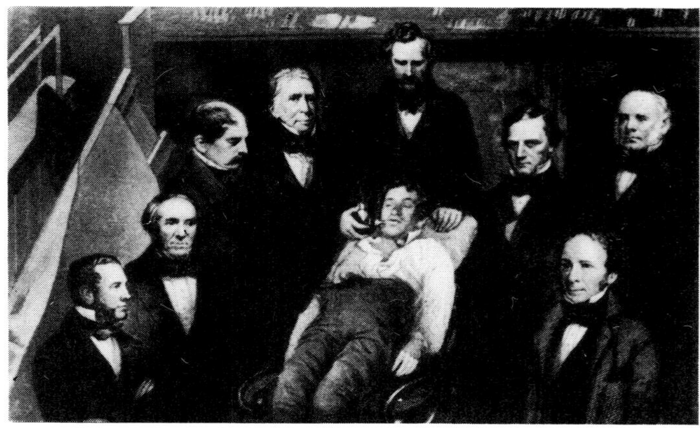

Item 5

For the reasons outlined in the introduction, the putative scene at the first use of nitrous oxide by Horace Wells (1815–48) in his office in 1844, and the first use of ether by William Morton (1819–68) at the Massachusetts General Hospital in 1846, have been the subject of a large number of differing representations: in words, photographs, oil paintings, engravings, dioramas and even film (*The Great Moment*, 1944). Many of the representations in circulation are third and fourth hand copies. Several replicas of Morton's inhaler have also been made, but even this apparently innocuous activity has provoked differences of opinion over the design of the apparatus he originally used (Duncum, 1947: 105–9, 552–61; Thomas, 1975: 9–10). The priority approach to the history of anaesthesia has customarily represented its discovery as a series of individual initiatives, often extending back to antiquity. Paradoxically, the sum total of this activity has often been described in terms of a biological process, usually evolution.

WILLIAM MORTON (1819–68)

3. OIL PAINTING 'The first use of ether in dental surgery, 1846, by W.T.G. Morton'. Oil-painting on canvas by Ernest Board (1877–1934), c. 1912. Commissioned by Henry Wellcome (1853–1936) through C.J.S. Thompson (1862–1943), the first curator of his collections. This was presumably intended to represent the operation in Morton's dental surgery, September 30, 1846 (Duncum, 1947: 105). 915 x 610 mm.

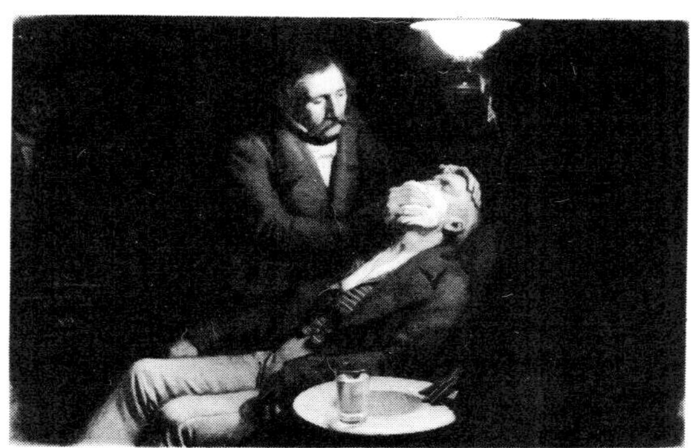

4. DAGUERREOTYPES Photographs of two of the three extant daguerreotypes taken to show the early use of ether at the Massachusetts General Hospital. Taken by Southworth and Hawes, 1847, (Burns, 1983: 1262; Duncum 1947: 117).
    (a) A male patient
    (b) A female patient
At some point the first of these two pictures became a model for later representations of the 'first operation'. (Originals in The Fogg Art Museum, Harvard University)

5. ENGRAVING of 'Wm. T.G. Morton M.D. Boston, making the first public demonstration of etherization', in Nathan P. Rice, *Trials of a public benefactor, as illustrated in the discovery of etherization*, New York, Pudney and Russell, 1859, f. p. 92. The book was a defence of Morton. The representation seems to have been based on the daguerreotype (a) above.

6. PHOTOGRAVURE A representation described as 'The first public demonstration of surgical anaesthesia', in *The semi-centennial of anaesthesia October 16, 1846–October 16, 1896*, Boston, Massachusetts General Hospital, 1897. A photogravure of a picture which seems to have been based on the daguerreotype (a) above.

7. POSTCARD of a diorama, described as 'The first surgical operation performed with a general anaesthetic', possibly copied from the photogravure described above. Produced for WHMM, c. 1955.

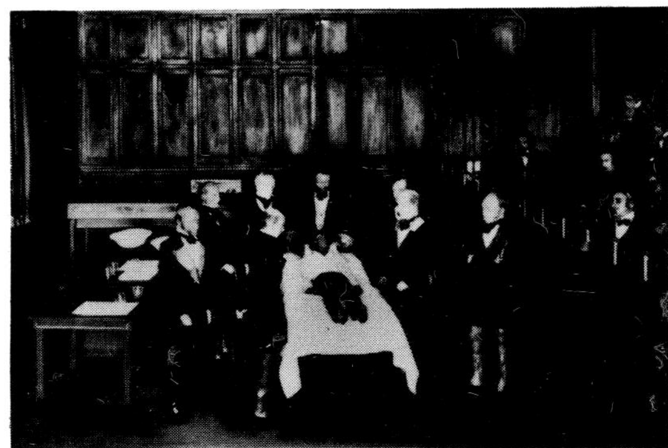

8. REPRODUCTION OF A PAINTING by Robert Hinckley (1853–1941), representing the first operation under ether, showing Morton administering the vapour. The patient is seated, not supine as in the daguerreotypes. *Scientific American*, 1985, *252* (4): 95. (Original painting in the Countway Library of Medicine, Boston)

9. GREAT MOMENTS Parke Davis and Company, *Great moments in medicine, stories by George A. Bender, paintings by Robert A. Thom*, Detroit, Northwood Institute Press, 1966. 'Conquerors of Pain', p. 185. A reproduction of a painting by Robert A. Thom representing the first use of ether by Morton. This picture seems to have been based on Hinckley's representation.

10. DISCOVERY Laird W. Nevius, *The discovery of modern anaesthesia. By whom was it made?*, New York, George W. Nevius, 1894. Nevius claimed this was the "first and only impartial, unprejudiced and fully illustrated publication" on the history of anaesthesia (Preface).

11. REPLICA of Morton's Ether Inhaler
c. 1945
A globular glass flask, connected to a glass mouthpiece via a brass cylinder with leather inspiratory and expiratory flap valves. A replica constructed for the Massachusetts General Hospital, owners of the inhaler claimed to have been used by W.T.G. Morton on October 16, 1846, for presentation to WHMM in 1946. A trademark for 'Pyrex' is onlaid at the neck of the flask.
190 x 292 x 153 mm. A625379

ANCIENT ANAESTHETICS

12. GREEK MESMERISM George Foy, *Anaesthetics, ancient and modern*, London, Baillière, Tindall & Cox, 1889. Foy's history began with "Mesmeric treatment not unknown to the Greeks" and finished with a review of the contemporary literature.

13. WELLCOME *Anaesthetics antient and modern*, Burroughs Wellcome & Co., London, 1907, containing a catalogue of Wellcome products. Historical essay by C.J.S. Thompson. An advertising booklet produced by the Company, for the annual meeting of the British Medical Association in Exeter, 1907. (WFA)

14. WELLCOME Paperbound version of *Anaesthetics antient and modern*, described in the previous entry, without the catalogue. (WFA)

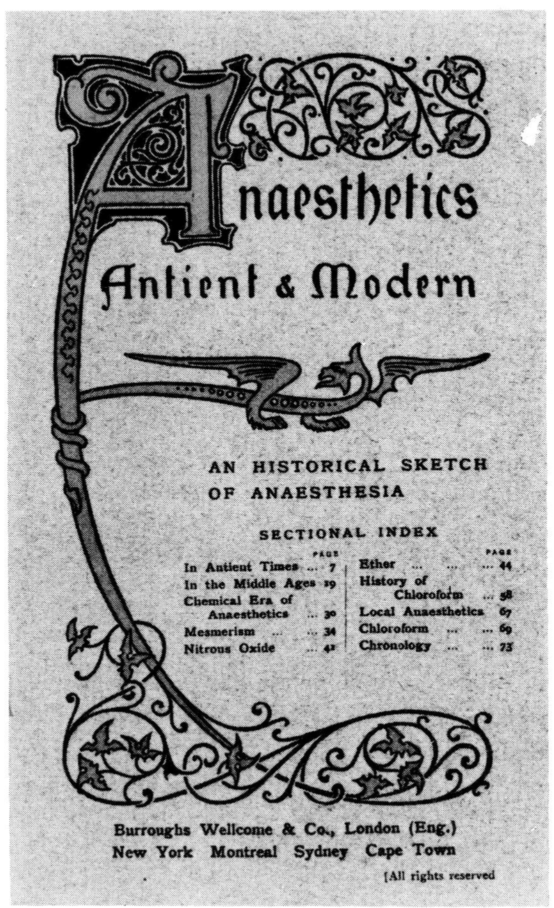

EVOLUTION

15. OBSTETRICS Andrew M. Claye, *The evolution of obstetric analgesia*, London, Oxford University Press, 1939. With the signature of Grantly Dick Read (1890–1959), 1939, on the fly-leaf. Read, a doctor and an early proponent of 'natural' childbirth, opposed anaesthesia except in abnormal deliveries.

16. ANAESTHESIA M.H. Armstrong Davison, *The evolution of anaesthesia*, Altrincham, John Sherratt & Son, 1965. A work "intended as a scientific and factual counterblast to the many romantic and largely fictional 'histories' of anaesthesia" (Preface).

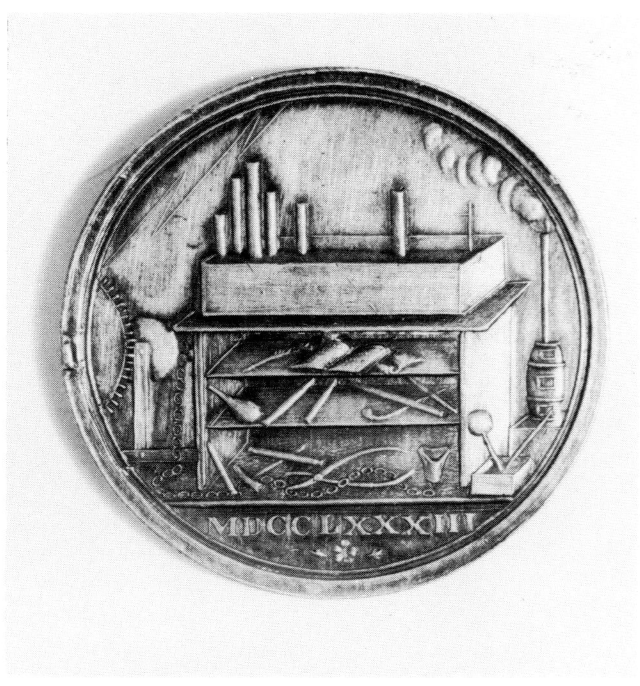

Item 17

An historical industry, related to the representation of the use of anaesthetics by Wells and Morton, has been the uncovering of precursors. A conventional starting point has been eighteenth century gas chemistry and, more particularly, the work of Joseph Priestley (1733–1804), Thomas Beddoes (1760–1808) and Sir Humphry Davy (1778–1829). Two figures have frequently been used to establish priorities: Crawford W. Long (1815–78) in America and Henry Hill Hickman (1800–30) in Britain. Although Hickman's experiments were familiar to nineteenth century authors (Buxton, 1888: 3), he was first investigated in detail by C.J.S Thompson (1862–1943), who worked for Sir Henry Wellcome (1853–1936). Thompson located the only known copy of the printed pamphlet in which Hickman described his experiments, together with an earlier manuscript draft. Thompson and other employees of Wellcome also collected various articles that had belonged to Hickman, and they were shown at exhibitions mounted by Wellcome in 1913 and 1930. The latter was produced to coincide with the centenary of Hickman's death. Works on precursors, such as Thompson's on Hickman, often use the metaphor of 'pioneer' (see below).

JOSEPH PRIESTLEY (1733–1804)

17. MEDAL of Joseph Priestley
1783 By J.G. Hancock
Silver medal, with R. profile bust inscribed 'Josephus Priestley/I.G. Hancock F.' *on obverse. On reverse*, chemical equipment. *In exergue* MDCCLXXXIII (see Brown, 1980: 59, no. 251). 1783 was Priestley's fiftieth year.
diameter 36 mm. A114795

18. COMMEMORATIVE MEDAL of Joseph Priestley
1804–1810 By T. Halliday
White metal medal, *on obverse*, L. profile bust of Priestley, *on a wide border around*, a list of his associations with learned societies. *On reverse*, an account of his life and works and the striking of the medal by his congregation after his death, *in exergue*, 'Unitarian Chapel, Birmingham' (see Brown, 1980: 138, no. 563).
diameter 51 mm. A129788

19. PLAQUE of Priestley
1777–1875
Oval, jasper ware plaque with profile bust of Priestley by John Flaxman (1755–1826) on a blue ground, by Wedgwood. A previous exhibition label: 'Joseph Priestley, FRS/ (The discoverer of oxygen)/ 1733–1804', is nailed to the gilded wooden frame.
328 x 266 mm. A639444

HENRY HILL HICKMAN (1800–30)

20. OIL PAINTING on canvas of Henry Hill Hickman. Copy commissioned by Wellcome through C.J.S. Thompson from an unknown artist, 1912, after the original portrait of c. 1830, also by an unidentified painter. Painted to hang among the Hickman memorabilia in WHMM, 1913. In 1912 the original was in the hands of Hickman's descendant, Mrs H.C. Bettridge. It is now in the possession of descendants of Hickman in Australia (Smith, 1970).
762 x 635 mm.

21. WATERCOLOUR of H.H. Hickman by Richard T. Cooper (*fl.* 1912–1930), 1912. Commissioned by Wellcome through C.J.S. Thompson, to illustrate Hickman's account of his experiments (Burgess, 1973: Ad. 21).
590 x 474 mm.

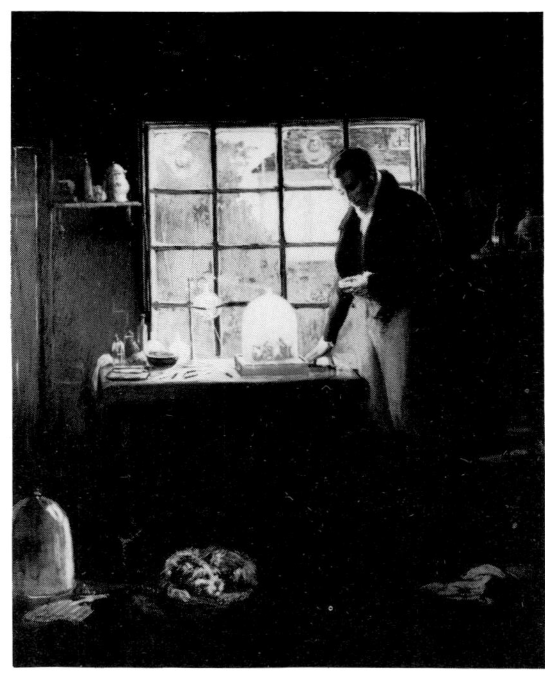

22. WAISTCOAT belonging to Henry Hill Hickman
1820–30
Satin-fronted, cotton-backed, black waistcoat, embroidered with blue floral pattern, mended in parts.
470 x 365 mm. A79271

23. DOORPLATE of Henry Hill Hickman
c. 1825
Brass, engraved and picked out in black: 'HICK-MAN'.
248 x 128 mm. A645118

24. POSTCARDS
(a) Postcard, postmarked February 5, 1912, from Blanche Thompson to C.J.S. Thompson (no relation) at Easley Mews, Wigmore St., London.
"Dear Sir, I am sending the pamphlet and visiting card by registered letter tomorrow Feb. 6th".
This refers to the only known copy of Hickman's pamphlet *A letter on suspended animation*, Ironbridge, W. Smith, 1824
(b) Postcard, postmarked Birmingham, March 14, 1930, to Mr. Malcolm, Wellcome Museum, 54 Wigmore Street, London.
"H.H.H. – I have received your letters saying pestle & mortar arrived safely. This you will see is a view of Ludlow. You may like to put it with the other views. I believe his house can be seen". The pestle and mortar were not Hickman's but belonged to his son in law, F. Falconer Thompson.
(c) Postcard showing a view of Ludlow, no postage stamp, no address, stamped "Received 17 March 1930".

"H.H.H. – From B.E. Thompson, Moseley. The cross I have put over the door I believe was number 9, Broadgate, where uncle William Thompson practised as a medical man before he went to London and H.H. Hickman before him".
Blanche Thompson (1856?–1941) was Hickman's granddaughter and daughter of F. Falconer Thompson. (b) and (c) were postcards to L.W.G. Malcolm (1888–1946) conservator of WHMM. The correspondence refers to Hickman family items. (Originals and other correspondence in WMSM and WIA)

25. PHOTOGRAPH by J. Ball, Kidderminster with accompanying inscription, "Represents eldest Grandson (Dr. F.H. Thompson of Hereford) and two great grandchildren of H.H. Hickman". From the Hickman memorabilia, collected by Malcolm. (WMSM)

26. EXHIBITION *Souvenir Henry Hill Hickman Centenary Exhibition*, London, The Wellcome Foundation Ltd., 1930, Preface. The Preface records that Wellcome's investigations revealed "certain unrecorded documents relating to Hickman's part in the History of Anaesthesia". An annotation by Thompson in the margin reads "The documents were not revealed in investigations they were discovered accidentally by me". (WIA)

27. PROGRAMME of a service at St. Mary the Virgin, Bromfield "at the Time of the Restoration of the Grave and the Unveiling of a Tablet in Memory of Henry Hill Hickman" April 5, 1930. (WIA)

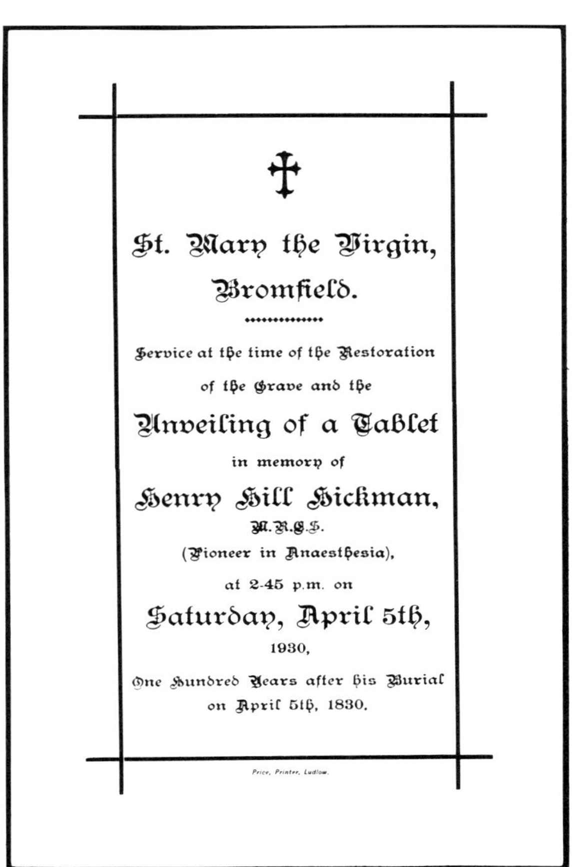

28. OFFPRINT C.J.S. Thompson 'Henry Hill Hickman, M.R.C.S., an English pioneer of anaesthesia'. Described as "Reprinted from the *BRITISH MEDICAL JOURNAL*, April 13th, 1912". The original article was actually entitled 'Henry Hill Hickman. A forgotten pioneer of anaesthesia', (Communicated from the Wellcome Historical Medical Exhibition Research) (*BMJ*, 1912, *i*: 843–5). It was initialled C.J.S.T. The 'reprint' was probably made in 1916.

29. HICKMAN *ET AL.* F.F. Cartwright, *The English pioneers of anaesthesia*, Bristol, John Wright & Sons Ltd., 1952.

CRAWFORD W. LONG (1815–78)

30. PHOTO-MECHANICAL PRINT of Crawford Long after a medallion by Robert Tait McKenzie (1867–1938), 1912.
This is probably a souvenir of the unveiling of a bronze medallion in the medical building of the University of Pennsylvania on March 30, 1912 (Freeman, 1964: 162–3; for speeches made on that occasion see Taylor, 1925: 416–8).
Tait McKenzie was a physician and sculptor who, from 1904, was Professor of Physical Education at the University of Pennsylvania.
sheet 355 x 279 mm.

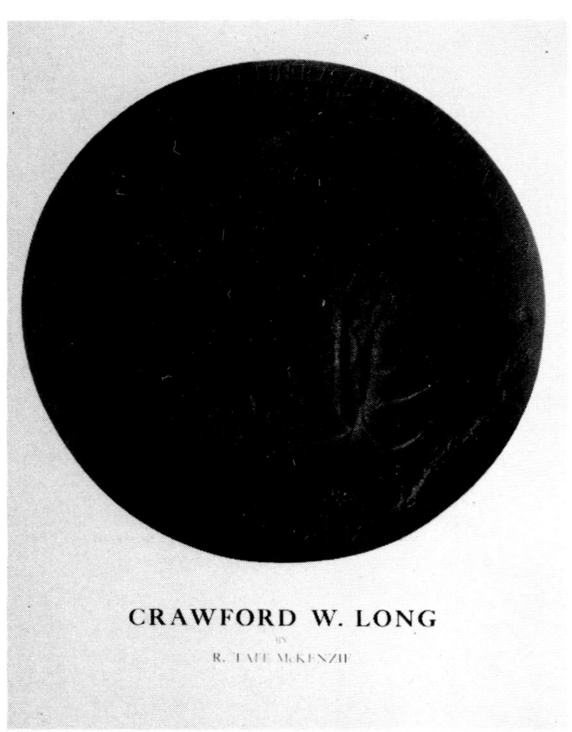

31. PHOTOGRAPH of a tintype (c. 1860), said to be of Crawford Long. It is evidently a staged demonstration of Long's use of ether in 1842. Long could be either the older man, if the demonstration was not staged until c. 1860, or the younger man if the picture is a copy made from an earlier daguerreotype. (Original in the Historical Collections at the University of Texas Health Science Center at San Antonio)

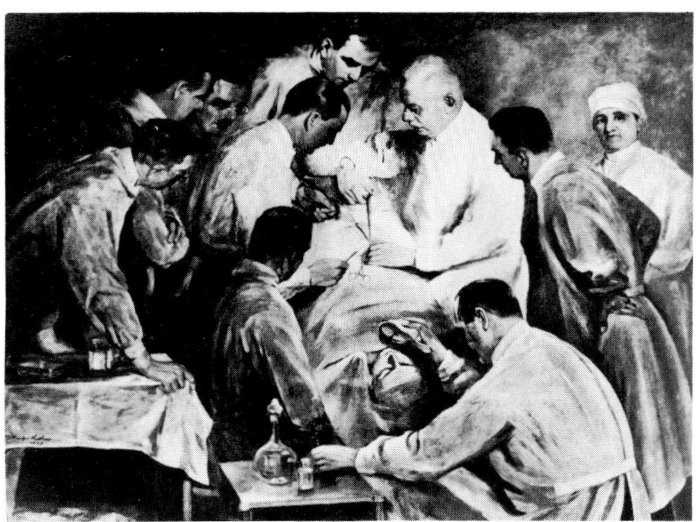

The history of anaesthesia has been repeatedly celebrated since the mid-nineteenth century; 1896 and 1946 in particular were dates marked by elaborate representations of anaesthetic history. This celebratory tradition has usually concentrated on the initiatives of individuals, Sir James Young Simpson (1811–70) figuring large in the British context. Representations of such individuals have been produced in a wide variety of forms and materials. Where possible, celebrations have also displayed artefacts which were associated with historical figures.

Item 48

SIR JAMES YOUNG SIMPSON (1811–70)

32. DRAWING Sir James Young Simpson and friends. Pen and ink drawing, heightened with white on artist's board. Authorship and date unknown. Provenance unknown before its accession in 1932. It represents Simpson's discovery of the anaesthetic properties of chloroform (for a textual description of the subject see Comrie, 1932, vol. 2: 601).
207 x 367 mm.

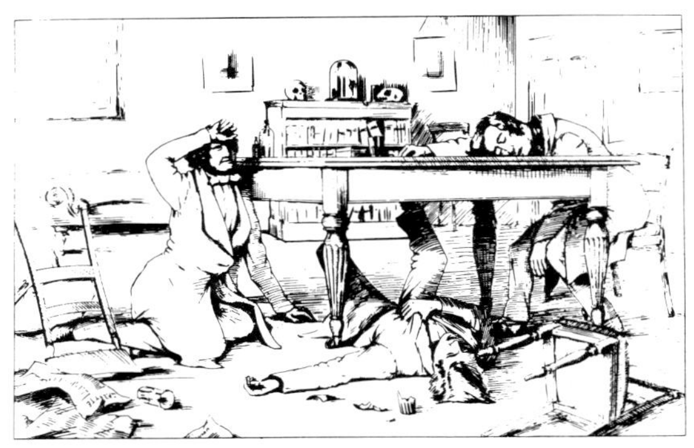

33. PHOTOGRAPH of a diorama representing the discovery of the anaesthetic effects of chloroform by Simpson. The diorama (not located) was made for WHMM, c. 1955. It was based on the drawing described in the previous entry.

34. STAINED GLASS WINDOW
c. 1890
One of four leaded glass window panels from the house of a medical practitioner in North London, said to depict James Young Simpson. A second panel apparently shows Edward Jenner (1749–1823), the remaining two bear designs incorporating serpents.
452 x 452 mm.   A639481

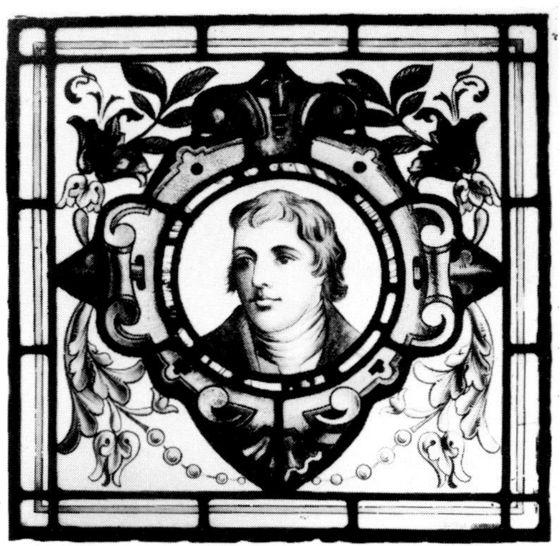

35. LITHOGRAPH portrait of Simpson by Frederick Schenck (*fl.* 1860s–80s), Edinburgh, after a drawing from life by James Archer (1824–1904). This impression is undated, but is probably of about the same date as another impression in the Wellcome Institute dated 1848. The other impression bears the legend "Dr. J.Y. Simpson. Professor of Midwifery in the University of Edinburgh" (Burgess, 1973: 2740.1).
285 x 233 mm.

36. OIL-PAINTING on cardboard of Simpson. Anon., date unknown. An enlarged copy of the lithograph described above, probably painted after World War One. Offered for sale at Foster's auction house, London, 25 November 1931, lot 151, and bought by Wellcome. A newspaper cutting pasted to the back of the board, 'A wonderful discovery', describes Simpson's discovery of the anaesthetic effects of chloroform and its benefits.
406 x 340 mm.

37. PHOTOGRAPH of a bust of J.Y. Simpson by W. Wallace (Original not located).

CENTENNIAL

38. PRINTED POSTER advertising the exhibition, 'Centenary of Anaesthesia' held at the WHMM, 183-193 Euston Road, London NW1, 1946. Open daily to the public. Admission free. (WIA)

THE WELLCOME HISTORICAL MEDICAL MUSEUM

CENTENARY OF ANAESTHESIA

Exhibition illustrating the

HISTORY OF SURGICAL ANAESTHESIA

at the

WELLCOME HISTORICAL MEDICAL MUSEUM

183-193. Euston Road. N.W.1

Open Daily to the Public

10.0 a.m. — 5.0 p.m. : Saturdays. 10.0 a.m. — 12 noon

until December 31st 1946

ADMISSION FREE

39. PRINTED INVITATION to A. G. Levy (1866-1954) to attend the opening of the exhibition, October 16, 1946, by Lord Moran, President of the Royal College of Physicians of London. (WIA)

40. PHOTOGRAPHS stamped 'Times Copyright', taken at the opening of the exhibition.
(a) Dr. E. Ashworth Underwood (1899–1980) shows Lord and Lady Moran Robert Liston's operating table. Underwood was Director of WHMM.
(b) Lady Moran cuts the tape at the opening. (WIA)

41. PHOTOGRAPHS of J.T. Clover (1825–82)
(a) The administration of chloroform.
(b) Filling the reservoir bag of his chloroform apparatus, 1862.
Frequently reproduced representations which were copied for the Wellcome centennial exhibition.
(From originals in the Nuffield Department of Anaesthetics, Oxford, presented by Mary Clover)

42. CLOVER'S BAG for use with his Chloroform Apparatus
c. 1870
A gusseted bag of impermeable fabric, with a wooden collar to connect with tubing, and two metal rings to take tapes on its upper edge. Clover's chloroform apparatus, exhibited in 1862 (Traer, 1862), filled the bag with a four and a half percent chloroform vapour in air mixture, prior to the administration of the anaesthetic. Exhibited at the centennial.
570 x 830 mm. (empty). A600332

43. CLOVER'S BAG for Nitrous Oxide Gas
c. 1868
Fabric-covered rubber bag with two loops of tape attached to the upper edge. A collar is missing from the 30 mm. aperture.
This is alleged to be from Clover's original apparatus for nitrous oxide anaesthesia. The bag was carried on his back during the administration (for a description of its use, see Duncum, 1947: 285–287).
790 x 535 mm. (empty). 1983–881/108

44. PHOTOGRAPH of a portrait mask of John Snow (1813–58) made by Mrs Ruth Poynter, 1946. Presumably the mask was displayed in the centennial exhibition. Noel Poynter (1908–79) was at this time Deputy Librarian of what was then the Wellcome Historical Medical Library (Original not located).

45. SPECIAL ISSUE 'Centenary of Anaesthesia', *British Medical Bulletin*, 1946, *4*: 81–164.

COLLECTING

46. BOOKPLATE of A. Charles King (1888–1966), 1946, in Edward William Murphy, *Chloroform; its properties and safety in childbirth*, London, Walton and Maberly, 1855. King was an instrument maker and collector of historical anaesthetic apparatus and texts (Thomas, 1970; Idem, 1975). (RSM)

47. PHOTOGRAPH of an advertisement by A. Charles King, inviting anaesthetists to hand him their unwanted books and journals instead of donating them directly to salvage. *British Journal of Anaesthesia*, 1942, *18*: f. contents. King presented his collection to the Association of Anaesthetists in 1953.

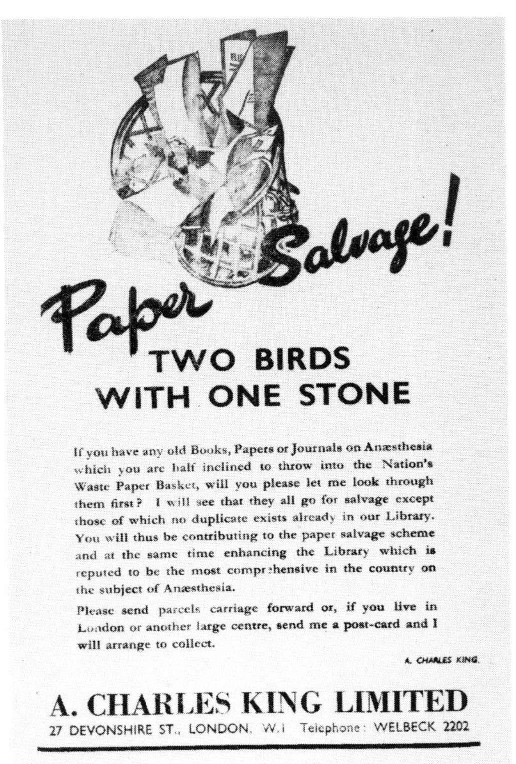

PICTURING SURGERY

48. PRINT 'Geheimrat Bumm bei einer Operation'. Photo-mechanical reproduction of a painting by Reinhard Huebner, 1925. Published by Gustav Schauer, Berlin.
Nine surgeons and a sister surround the operating table, on which a female patient is lying. *To r*, Ernst Bumm (1848–1925) holding forceps over operation site; *facing him*, his first assistant Kurt Warnekros (1882–1949); *at head of patient*, Erich Fischer? (1893–1975) lifting a Schimmelbusch mask from patient's face; *to l of him*, Paul Sippel? (b. 1882) At head of pyramidal group Karl Ruge (b. 1885); *to r of the professor*, Paul Schäfer? (1881–1965). Possibly the figures identified here as Fischer and Schäfer should be transposed (Leibbrand, 1965; and information from Dr. Renate Burgess from correspondence with Professor W. Hoffmann-Axthelm and Dr. Walter Warnekros, Berlin, 25.4.1977, and with Professor B. Sarembe, Dresden, 27.6.1977).
414 x 557 mm.

49. PRINT 'Operation in Progress', a representation of a modern surgical scene, "Painted for Imperial Chemical Industries Limited by Anna Zinkeisen" and published in *'Trilene' in analgesia and anaesthesia*, Manchester, Imperial Chemical Industries, 1949. A booklet produced by ICI to describe their trichlorethylene product, 'Trilene'. (Loaned by Dr. David Wilkinson)

50. OIL PAINTING on canvas with key on panel, 'The Incision: a tribute to medical research', by Richard Bannister, n.d. [1970s]. The painting shows a modern surgical operation surrounded by the heroes who have contributed to medicine. Morton is shown on the extreme right with his inhaler next to a gas and oxygen machine. Mr Bannister was on the staff of St. Mary's Hospital, Paddington, when he painted the picture.
canvas and key 1070 x 1100 mm.

CASE 4: IMAGES OF ANAESTHESIA: PUBLIC PERCEPTIONS

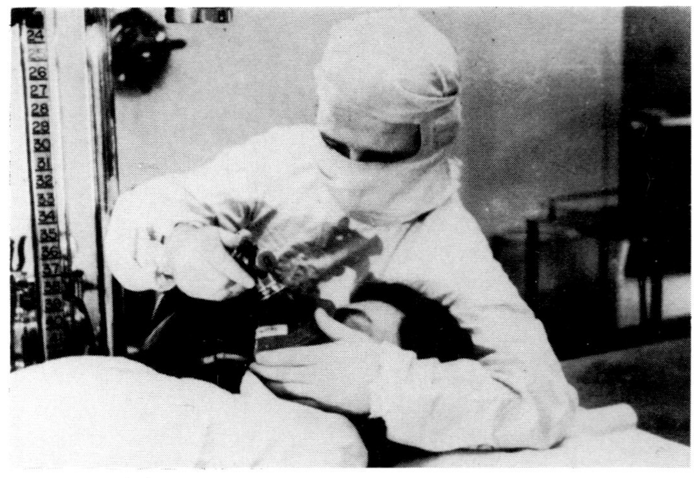

Item 54(b)

One consequence of the emphasis on individual innovation in the history of anaesthetics has been the neglect of the place of anaesthesia in culture generally. There are no studies, for example, of public perceptions of inhalational anaesthesia in the early years of its use, or of how the meanings of pain were changed in response to its employment (but see Pernick, 1985). Anaesthesia has also appeared in the public arena associated with things other than surgery. Almost from its first employment and up to the present day, anaesthesia, in fact and fiction, has been associated with crime, notably rape, theft and kidnapping. The question of who should use anaesthetic agents has been much debated, occasionally by Parliament and the press. This issue has usually involved the familiar balancing of individual rights versus professional expertise. Anaesthetics and antivivisection were also contentious areas in the late nineteenth century. In Britain, the 1876 Cruelty to Animals Act included a section which regularized the use of anaesthetics in animal experiments.

THE PRESS

51. CARTOON depicting 'Wonderful effects of ether in a case of scolding wife', *Punch*, February 6, 1847, p. 60. The cartoon showed the persecuted husband enjoying an ether-induced "beautiful dream" oblivious to his "scolding wife".

52. PHOTOGRAPH of *Punch*, August 14, 1847, p. 60, 'Ether and humming bees', reporting the use of ether to render bees inactive in order to procure their honey.

53. PHOTOGRAPH of the words of a song to be sung to an air from 'The Beggar's Opera', from *The Illustrated London News*, Jan. 30, 1847. Reprinted in *The Lancet*, 1946, *ii*: 611.

> How happy could I be with Æther
> Were mesmeric charmers away,
> But while they perplex me together
> The Devil a word can I say.
> Sing Robinson, Thomson, and Cooper,
> Fol Lol de Rol, Lol de Rol, Lay
> There's nothing like Æther and Stupor
> For making a hospital gay.

54. PHOTOGRAPHS of 'A street accident and what follows'. A photostory from *Picture Post*, January 7, 1939, pp. 18–22.

    (a) The story, with short captions, followed the history of Tom who, after being knocked down on a London street, was admitted to St. Bartholomew's Hospital. The anaesthetist figured prominently in one of the pictures.

    (b) Photograph of one of the episodes in the photostory described above, 'The anaesthetist watches for the slightest change'. (Copyright Hulton Picture Library)

55. PHOTOGRAPH of a part of a photostory in *Picture Post*, July 22, 1944, p. 11, 'A hospital for war nerves', entitled 'One of the treatments which help doctor and patient get at the truth'. The picture shows the doctor injecting a "narcotic".

MUSEUMS

56. CATALOGUE Nancy Knight, *Pain and its relief. An exhibition at the National Museum of American History*, Washington, D.C., Smithsonian Institution, 1983. "The exhibition, made possible by a grant from the American Society of Anesthesiologists, dramatically illustrates the progress that has been made in understanding and controlling pain" (Exhibition handout). (WMSM)

57. PHOTOGRAPH of a reconstruction described as "A state-of-the-art operating room for coronary bypass surgery [which] serves as a focal point in "Pain and Its Relief" " (Handout for the exhibition described above). (WMSM)

CRIME

58. THEFT John Snow, 'The alleged employment of chloroform by thieves', reprinted from the *London Medical Gazette*, February 22, 1850. Bound with three other papers on chloroform by Snow.

59. ROBBERY Photograph of the *Pharmaceutical Journal*, 1849–50, *9*: 393, 'Robbery by means of chloroform'.

60. RAPE Photograph of *The British Medical Journal*, 1877, *ii*: 708, 'Charge of rape under chloroform'.

61. RAPE Photograph of a passage from 'Attempted Rape under Anaesthetics', in Chapter XII, 'Medico-legal aspects of the administration of anaesthetics', in Dudley Wilmot Buxton, *Anaesthetics. Their uses and administration*, 4th ed., London, H.K. Lewis, 1907, p. 384.   Buxton discussed crime, consent, deaths, responsibility, illegal operations, poisoning, addiction and "insanity following the administration of anaesthetics".

ADDICTION

62. PHOTOGRAPH of *The British Medical Journal*, 1888, *i*: 1021, 'A victim to the chloroform habit'. The article described a woman who "would take a pint of chloroform in the day". The journal criticized "the laxity of some person or persons in selling chloroform to her".

63. PHOTOGRAPH of *The British Medical Journal*, 1890, *ii*: 885, an article by Ernest Hart, on 'Ether-drinking; its prevalence and results'. Hart described the practice as particularly prevalent in Ireland.

SELF PERCEPTIONS

64. ARTICLE 'The anaesthetist 1964', a representation of the anaesthetist's roles, *St. Bartholomew's Hospital Journal*, 1964, *68*: 302.

EXPERIMENTATION

65. ENGRAVING 'Vivisection', by Charles John Tomkins (b. 1847, worked c. 1876–c. 1894) after John McLure (or McClure) Hamilton (1853–1936), after a painting or drawing of 1882. The date of the original work and the artist's signature are reproduced in the bottom right corner.
Hamilton's original was exhibited in London in the autumn of 1885 bearing the title, 'Vivisection – the last appeal'. It portrays an animal experimenter holding behind his back what is, presumably, a bottle of an anaesthetic, and facing a dog begging for mercy (Schupbach, 1987).
610 x 435 mm.

ADVERTISING

66. TRADE CARD 'The wonder of the age', advertising the use of "vitalized air for the extraction of teeth without pain" at Dr. Free's York Dental Parlors, 50 North George Street, York, Pennsylvania, n.d. (Loaned by Dr. Ben Z. Swanson Jr.)

PATIENT PERCEPTIONS

67. PHOTOGRAPH of J.F.B. Flagg, *Ether and chloroform*, Philadelphia, Lindsay and Blakiston, 1851, p. 110. Flagg described the case of an Irishwoman who consented to having ether administered "on being told she would suffer no pain, and would *probably* have an interview with her friends in the old country".

68. OIL PAINTING on canvas, 'On the periphery', by Pauline Annesley, date unknown (before 1980).
According to Mr. N. Asherson FRCS, who presented this picture to WHL, it shows "What the patient saw. The scene as visualised by the artist who regained consciousness during a gynaecological operation, but was still paralysed by the relaxant" (On patient awareness during operations see, *BMJ*, 1978, *i*: 48, 300; Hargrove, 1987).
695 x 450 mm.

CASE 5: ANAESTHESIA AND THE VICTORIANS

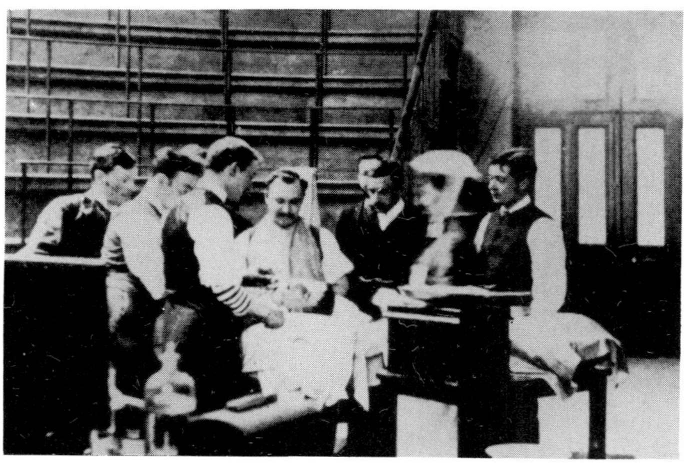

Item 71

The events surrounding the communication of Morton's success with ether to Britain, and Robert Liston's (1794–1847) trial of the 'Yankee dodge' at University College Hospital, London on December 21, 1846, have been well documented by historians. Perhaps predictably, a claim has been made that another hospital was in fact the site of the earliest British use of anaesthesia for major surgery – the Dumfries and Galloway Infirmary – over 300 miles from London and a stop for the paddle steamer which apparently carried the news of Morton's discovery to this country (Sykes, 1960: 150–9; Ellis, 1976). Equally well covered has been the hurried construction of the earliest inhalers and the various recorded instances where ether was first used for dental and surgical operations at the turn of 1846 (Duncum, 1947; Sykes, 1960: 48–76). Much less work, however, has been done on the way in which anaesthesia was subsequently incorporated into the everyday practice of Victorian surgery – who gave and who received which anaesthetic agents and by which means.

Some statistics on the use of anaesthetics were compiled and published from Victorian hospital practice. An Assistant Surgeon to the Eye Department of Guy's Hospital, London, recorded in 1870 that, between 1862–69, 3,483 patients had received an anaesthetic there. By far the greater number (3,224) were given chloroform. The remainder received nitrous oxide (26), ether (3) or bichloride of methylene, with or without chloroform (230). The operations had mostly lasted "two to three minutes", and no fatalities had occurred, although "a feeling of unsafety was experienced at the administration of the anaesthetic in every case" (Bader, 1870: 100). We have as yet, however, rather few insights into practice outside London and outside hospitals. Much major surgery was, until the end of the century, performed in the homes of wealthier patients. Early texts on anaesthetic agents, such as A.E. Sansom's (1838–1907) *Chloroform: its action and administration* are occasionally a source of considerable detail regarding the practicalities of anaesthesia (Sansom, 1865). They reveal a world where the intending anaesthetist was obliged to apply a battery of chemical tests, involving agents such as egg white and sulphuric acid, to ascertain the presence of dangerous impurities in the chloroform he was about to use, where he was not perturbed if, under anaesthesia, a sailor patient sang his sea songs, or a young girl a hymn "correctly, word for word and note for note" throughout the whole course of a surgical operation, and where "sympathising relatives" who "happen to be in the room at the time of an operation" required his attentions as much as did the patient (Ibid.: 19, 29, 31). Sansom's text also clearly reveals one much overlooked aspect of the introduction of anaesthetic agents – the great expectations of their therapeutic, as well as anaesthetic, properties. "The use of vapour-medicines, whether for ... (anaesthesia), or for the general treatment of diseased conditions, is in its infancy as a science ... doubtless the results will be of never-ending value" (Ibid.: 35, see also *Anaesthesia and Innovation*).

It is not only the practical details of administration, in what must have been thousands of unrecorded and presumably uneventful anaesthetics that are hard to find. It is equally difficult to assess the effects of anaesthesia on surgical practice. Some authors have addressed this issue, suggesting that surgical mortality rose in the years immediately following the introduction of anaesthesia, with surgeons overreaching their capabilities in both the extent of the operations they performed and the selection of suitable patients. However, a recent reappraisal by Pernick seems to show that, in America at least, this was not the case (Pernick, 1985: 217–21). Rising surgical mortality can as justifiably be blamed, he suggests, on factors such as industrialisation, as on the use of anaesthesia (see also Hamilton, 1982).

Pernick's work also shows that, as late as the 1870s, by no means all patients undergoing even major surgery received an anaesthetic. Certain groups – children, and women – usually did, although the very young and the very old were sometimes considered too frail. Male patients had only a one in three chance of receiving anaesthesia for limb amputation at the Pennsylvania Hospital between 1853 and 1862 (Pernick, 1985: 192–3).

SURGERY

69. PHOTOGRAPH showing the administration of an inhalational anaesthetic, almost certainly chloroform, at the Royal Infirmary, Edinburgh, c. 1900. (From an original in the Royal Infirmary, Edinburgh)

70. PHOTOGRAPH showing an operation in progress at St. Bartholomew's Hospital, c. 1895.

71. PHOTOGRAPH showing the administration of an inhalational anaesthetic, probably chloroform, but possibly ether, by dropping the agent on to a face-mask, at St. Thomas's Hospital, 1889 (*St. Thomas's Hospital Gazette*, 1965, *63* (2): 72).

72. PHOTOGRAPH of *The British Medical Journal*, 1870, *i*: 100, showing statistics for anaesthetic administration at the Eye Department of Guy's Hospital.

ETHER INHALATION

73. TRACY'S ETHER INHALER
1847–8
A glass 'hookah', with ground glass stopper, designed to contain ether-saturated sponges. A brass stopcock joins the inhaler to fabric-covered, flexible tubing and, via a wooden connector and side-tube, to a mouthpiece (missing from this example).
In early 1847 Samuel John Tracy (1812/3–1901) of St. Bartholomew's Hospital, London, introduced his inhaler, "hookahs appearing to be the fashionable shape" *(Pharm. J.*, 'On the inhalation', 1846–7, *vi*: 357–8). It was intended largely for use in dental extractions. The side tube in this example was added to facilitate administration in recumbent patients. Within the year, Tracy, like many others, came to prefer an ether-soaked sponge alone, through which the patient could breathe more easily (Duncum, 1947: 146).
600 x 370 x 43 mm. A600331

74. HEDLEY'S ETHER INHALER
1847
A wooden bottle with removable base, containing cotton wool beneath a discoid inspiratory valve which divides the bottle into upper and lower compartments. A similar expiratory valve covers an aperture adjacent to the mouthpiece.
Dr. G.D. Hedley of Bedford (*fl.* 1838–49) designed this inhaler in 1847, (*Pharm. J.*, 'Dr. Hedley's ether inhaler', 1846–7; ibid., 'Ether inhaler of Dr. Hedley', 1847–8), originally to contain an ether-soaked sponge. Wood was used rather than glass in an attempt to avoid the freezing which occurred as ether vaporized. Its construction involved the use of mahogany, lignum vitae, cherry tree and boxwood. The inhaler does not seem to have been produced commercially.
183 x 74 x 74 mm. A87601

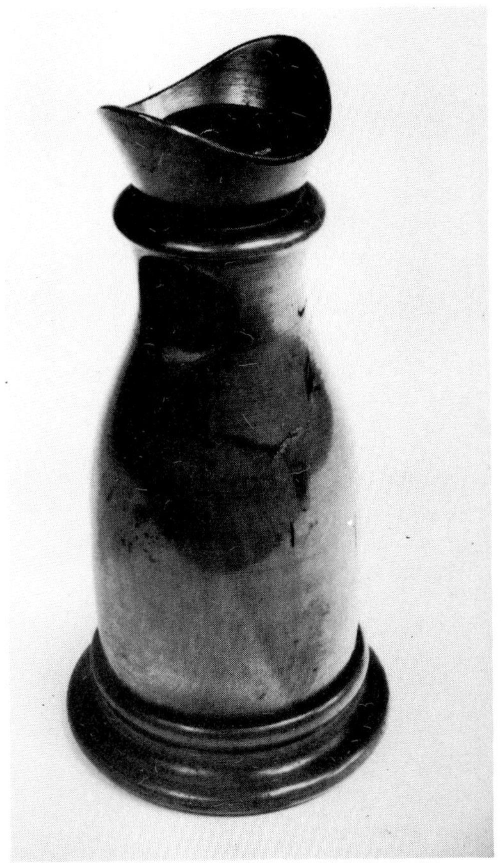

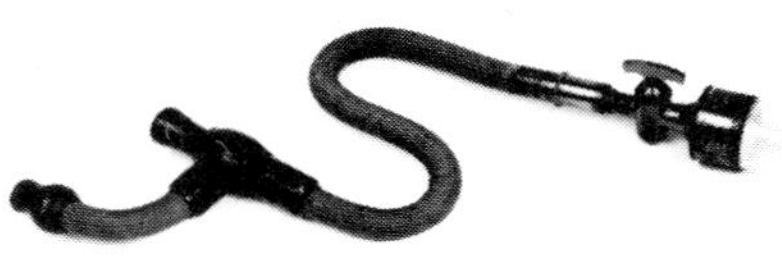

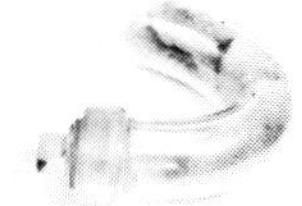

75. MORGAN'S ETHER INHALER
c. 1880
A leather-covered, double-walled, metal cone with a felt lining and chamois-lined facepiece.
An ether-soaked sponge was placed in the apex, adjacent to an air inlet valve. Exhaled air passed through a second valve into the cavity between the walls of the inhaler, to maintain its warmth. The air was then led away from the patient via a further valve and a length of tubing (missing from this example). A flared metal inlet for fresh air, which could be covered by the finger, perforates the upper surface of the cone. This is absent from Morgan's original description *(BMJ,* 'An ether inhaler', 1876).
John H. Morgan (1847–1924), house surgeon and subsequently surgical registrar at St. George's Hospital, London, introduced this alternative to the plain felt cone for the sake of the anaesthetist's comfort and pocket – it reduced the amount of ether vapour escaping into the room and the overall amount of ether required. According to Morgan's description, the original makers were Messrs. Blaise and Co., 67, St. James's Street, but the inhaler has not been found in any commercial catalogue. Resembling as it did the 'reckless' American method of giving ether, specialists may have disdained it. Buxton referred to the cone as a "contrivance largely used in America" (Buxton, 1888: 57) and, describing the method, stated: "This plan is not satisfactory" (Buxton, 1900: 126).
240 x 88 mm.   A55237

76. CLOVER'S PORTABLE REGULATING ETHER INHALER
1877–1920 *Mayer & Meltzer/LONDON. W.*
The inhaler consists of a domed, nickel-plated reservoir into which one and a half ounces of ether were poured via the filling tube. A water jacket to prevent excessive cooling partially surrounds the reservoir, which rotates on a metal tube running through its centre, connecting the facemask to the rubber bag (missing from this example). A system of opposing ports in the inner tube opens or closes as the chamber is rotated, allowing more or less air to pass out over the surface of the ether. This is indicated on an arbitrary, engraved scale of 1–2–3–F, by the pointer. J. T. Clover (1825–82) described this inhaler in 1877 (Clover, 1877). It was the first to incorporate a method of regulating the amount of ether inhaled and was designed to prevent admission of air, in what came to be known as the 'closed method' for ether. Together with Ormsby's inhaler (Ormsby, 1877) it was described in textbooks until the 1940s, in modified forms, for closed ether, and was supplied to the Royal Air Force at the outbreak of World War Two (Atkinson and Boulton, 1977: 1033). Clover himself used it little (Duncum, 1947: 344), but the numerous modifications indicate that others did. Like many innovations in anaesthesia, these modifications have been the subject of subsequent priority debates (Galley and King, 1948). This particular example incorporates a tap which allows the gas bag to be filled

with nitrous oxide (see Bond, 1884), but Clover's personal inhaler seems also to have included such a device (Atkinson and Boulton, 1977: 1034).
175 x 90 mm.   A625272

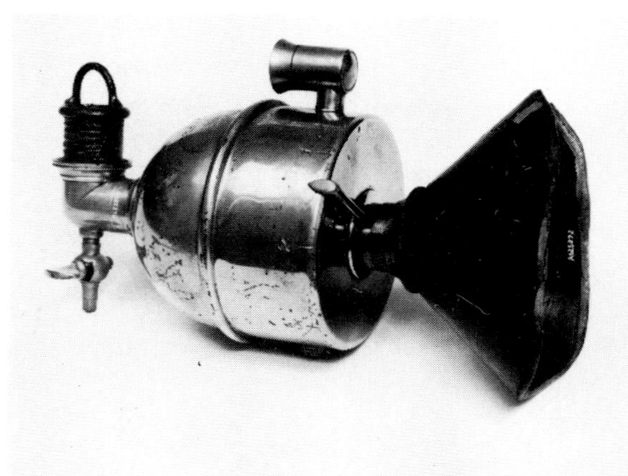

77. JULLIARD'S Ether Mask
1877–1900
Gauze covered wire frame, with waxed fabric outer cover and a "rosette" of flannel layers, on to which ether was poured, inside the apex of the dome.
The surgeon, Gustave Julliard (1836–1911) of Geneva began using ether after a chloroform fatality in 1877 (Duncum, 1947: 405). The waterproof outer cover of his mask prevented loss of ether vapour and necessitated a much larger frame than those designed for 'open' ether, to prevent asphyxiation. Although both Hewitt and Buxton frequently cited Julliard's work, especially on anaesthetic statistics, neither mentioned his mask, which seems not to have been widely used in Britain (Hewitt, 1901: 108; Buxton, 1900: 225).
120 x 170 x 145 mm.   1983–881/325

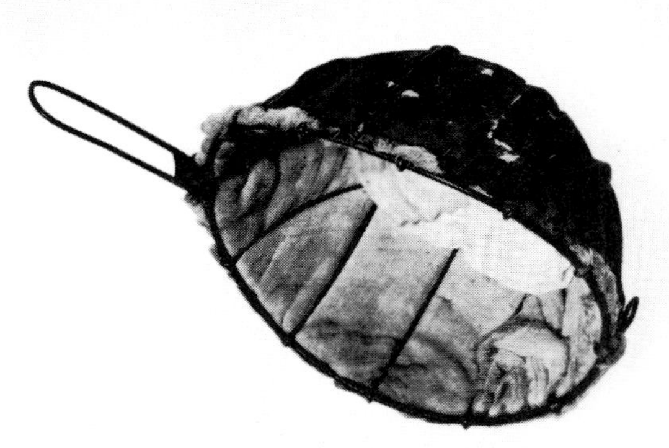

78. MONOGRAPH John Snow, *On the inhalation of the vapour of ether in surgical operations,* London, John Churchill, 1847.

CHLOROFORM INHALATION

79. SNOW'S CHLOROFORM INHALER (mask)
1848–70
Chamber and tube of Snow's chloroform inhaler
SAVIGNY & Co./ 67. St JAMES'S St.
A nickel-plated brass canister to contain cold water
and a second canister for chloroform. The internal
canister has air holes in the lid and contains a frame-
work of four metal strips to support blotting paper.
It attaches, by a bayonet fitting, to the cloth-covered,
flexible, metal tube. The facepiece (from a different
example) is of brass, lined with velvet. An inspiratory
valve, which can be swung away from an aperture, is
missing from the outer surface of the facepiece.
John Snow (1813–58) described this inhaler as a
means of delivering a four percent mixture of chloroform vapour in air, which he had found most suitable
for surgical anaesthesia (Snow, 1848: 179; *Pharm.
J.*, 'Dr. Snow's', 1847–8). Later descriptions include
a glass tube in the canister side to view the chloroform level (Snow, 1858: 81–5). The facemask, attributed to Francis Sibson (1814–76), was originally of
thin sheet lead, which Snow used because it excluded
air, previous inhalers having usually been fitted with
tubes, which dropped out of the patient's mouth and
"led generally to great awkwardness" (Snow, 1858:
83). The exclusion of air, however, was cited by Hewitt as the reason for this inhaler's decline (Hewitt,
1901: 315). In 1900, Buxton described it as having
"passed into desuetude", along with the chloroform
inhalers of Clover, Sansom and Squire (Buxton, 1900:
171).
mask 86 x 55 x 100 mm. A625286
canister 148 x 67 mm. A625273

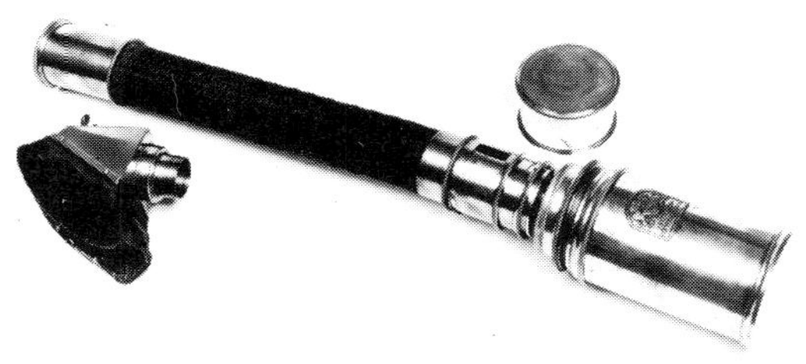

80. MONOGRAPH John Snow, *On chloroform and
other anaesthetics: their action and administration.
Edited with a memoir of the author by Benjamin W.
Richardson*, London, John Churchill, 1858. (RSM)

81. SANSOM'S modification of Snow's chloroform
inhaler
*1865–85 W. MATTHEWS 8. PORTUGAL St./
LINCOLN'S INN/LONDON*
A cylindrical, brass vaporizing chamber, containing a
roll of blotting paper to hold chloroform, is connected
via a pivoted, right-angled tube with adjustable air
inlet to a Snow/Sibson facepiece of leather and velvet
(see above). An expiratory flap valve on the facepiece
has been replaced.

Arthur Ernest Sansom (1838–1907), physician to the
London Hospital from 1874–1907, described this inhaler in 1865 (Sansom, 1865: 126–30). The water-
bath in Snow's original design was replaced with
gutta-percha insulation, (missing from this example)
and the flexible tube was dispensed with (on the *dis-
similarity* of this inhaler to Snow's, see Thomas, 1975:
68). Sansom was firmly of the opinion that an inhaler
should allow for extreme dilution of the chloroform
vapour, and a means of gradually increasing concentration, this entailing "very little sacrifice of time. Six
minutes are amply sufficient to induce the anaesthesia" (Sansom, 1865: 131).
160 x 60 x 140 mm. A600330

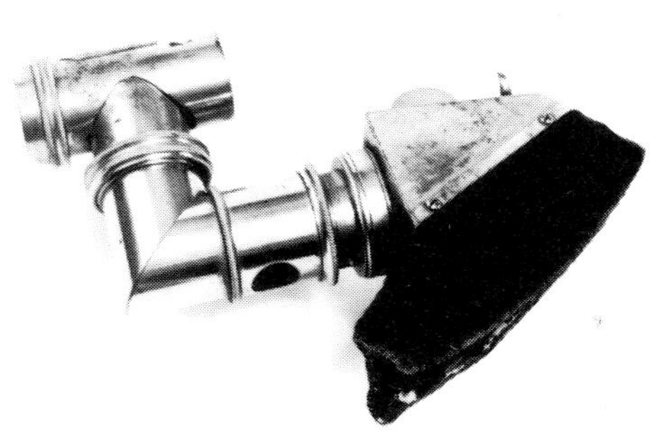

82. COATES'S modification of Snow's chloroform
inhaler
*1854–80 MATTHEWS/CAREY ST/LINCOLN'S
INN/LONDON.*
A spherical, brass vaporizing container, with air holes
in the lid, is connected to the rubber and brass facemask by an elbow tube. The mask has mica disc
inspiratory and expiratory valves.
The inventor seems likely to have been William Martin Coates (1812–85), surgeon at Salisbury Infirmary
who, in about 1850, was experimenting on the effects
of chloroform on frogs. He favoured Snow's apparatus
for his clinical work (Coates, 1851).
193 x 190 x 100 mm. A625413

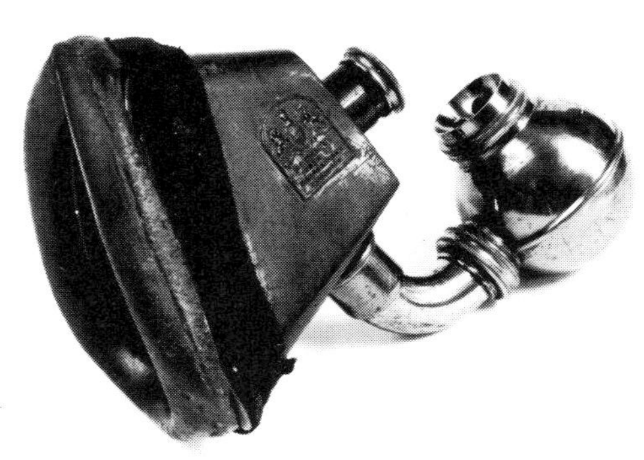

INHALERS

83. MADDOX inhaler
1847–1900
Plated copper holder for a chloroform-soaked sponge, with a perforated mouthpiece. A metal plate behind the mouthpiece prevents liquid chloroform being drawn into the mouth. The inhaler closely resembles that described by Coxeter, 23, Grafton Street, East, in 1847–8 (*Pharm. J.*, 'Chloroform inhaler', 1847–8, *vii*: 313) but attributed in a subsequent number to J.E. Maddox, 19, University St., University College (*Pharm. J.*, 1847–8, *vii*: 394).
75 x 55 x 72 mm. A600323

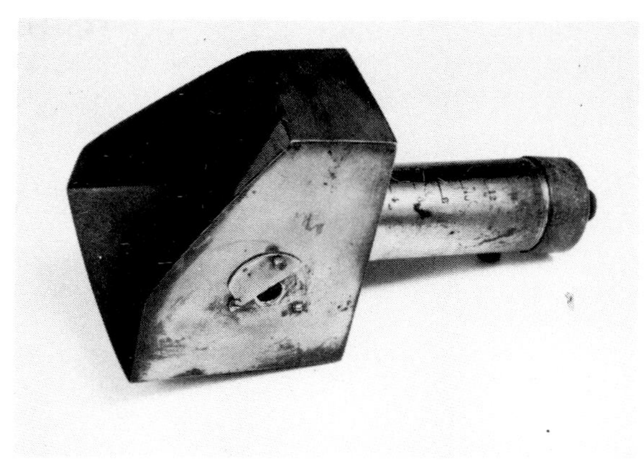

84. INHALER
1850–1900
A soldered tin box with brass fittings containing roughly cut pieces of felt, with a screw-on filler cap and detachable mask on opposite faces. A metal tube passes through the top of the box to connect with a rebreathing bag of animal membrane attached below. Square ports cut in the tube are rotated by means of a handle at the top to allow inhalation of fresh air, or of vapour from the rebreathing bag. The filler cap is inscribed, *Modèle Déposé, L.F.A.D.* No descriptions of this, apparently French, inhaler have been traced.
224 x 175 x 80 mm. A182596

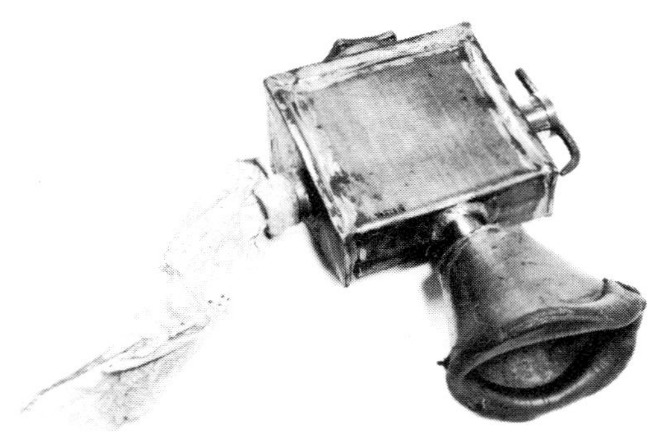

85. INHALER
1866–1900 *ARNOLD & SONS/35 & 36/WEST SMITHFIELD/LONDON*
A nickel-plated inhaler consisting of a box-like facepiece joined to a cylindrical chamber with a glass-lined, detachable metal inner tube, graduated 2–16, for liquid anaesthetic. A flannel cloth is stretched over a removable wire frame slotted into the facepiece, which has a variable air inlet. This inhaler does not appear in any of Arnold & Sons' trade catalogues.
190 x 92 x 108 mm. A625293

DROP BOTTLES

86. MILLS'S Chloroform Drop Bottle
1880–1932
Clear glass bottle with etched scale *0–14 DRMS*, with nipple-shaped metal stopper, screw cap and leather carrying case. Joseph Mills (d. 1893) was a full-time anaesthetist to St. Bartholomew's Hospital, London, between 1875–1893. Several special designs for anaesthetic drop bottles appeared in the late nineteenth century, but most textbooks did not bother to specify their use for open chloroform (e.g. Buxton, 1888: 78–9). From 1900, the convenience of drop bottles was stressed (Hewitt, 1901: 327) as was, increasingly, the necessity for those entering general practice to understand their use (Blomfield, 1922: 192). A substitute could be "easily and economically improvised with a four-ounce round-shouldered bottle and the stopper of a perfume bottle" (Luke, 1905: 78).
133 x 46 mm. 1983–881/856

87. THOMAS'S Chloroform Drop Bottle
1880–1932
Clear glass bottle with etched scale *0–16 DS*, the metal stopper containing a spring valve which can be arranged so as to close the bottle, to allow drops to escape as the spring is depressed, or to allow a steady stream. Recommending this design, Hewitt used about one drachm every four or five minutes in the first hour of anaesthesia – roughly a full bottle (Hewitt, 1901: 328).
131 x 45 mm. 1983–881/132

88. JACKSON'S Ether Drop Bottle
1913–32 *MAYER & MELTZER/LONDON*
Curved, pear-shaped, clear glass, 250 ml flask with metal filler cap and fine pouring tube with a tap to regulate air inlet, and hence dropping rate.
Douglas Jackson (d. 1942) stressed the convenient position of the anaesthetist's arm and hand allowed by this bottle (Jackson, 1913). It was not commonly recommended after about 1920.
260 x 49 mm. 1983–881/135

RETAIL ANAESTHETICS

89. SHOP ROUND for chloroform
1801–1910
Clear glass bottle with pourer and drip bowl, engraved *CHLOROFORM*. 1850–1900
238 x 86 mm. A660086

90. SHOP ROUND for ether
1801–1910
Clear glass bottle with painted gilt label *SP:AETHER:*.
200 x 74 mm. A632448

91. SHOP BOTTLE for chloroform
1862–3 *PATD SEP 23 1862 W.N. WALTON.*
Round, clear glass bottle with glass-fronted photo type label: SPIR./CHLOROF. W.N. Walton, an American company, supplied this bottle to J.A. Reid, Chemist, of Lochmaben, Dumfriesshire, in 1863. The patent refers to the glass-fronted label (Crellin and Scott, 1972: 45).
207 x 75 mm. A633829

92. CHLOROFORME ANESTHÉSIQUE
1850–1900 *A. Vicario/Pharmacien de 1ère Classe/17, Bould Haussmann (angle de la rue du Helder) Paris.*
Brown glass ampoule of chloroform "chimiquement pur" in cardboard cylinder with printed label.
179 x 32 mm. A56873

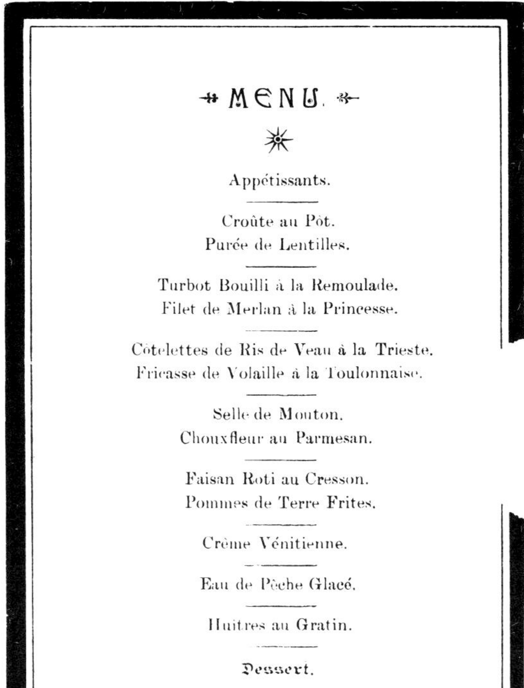

ETHER AND CHLOROFORM

93. AMERICA J.F.B. Flagg, *Ether and chloroform: their employment in surgery, dentistry, midwifery, therapeutics, etc.*, Philadelphia, Lindsay and Blakiston, 1851. An early American anaesthetic text.

94. BRITAIN Charles Kidd, *On aether and chloroform as anaesthetics*, 2nd ed., London, Renshaw, 1858. Inscribed "For the *Lancet* from the author" a book based, Kidd claimed, on "about 11,000 administrations".

THE PROFESSIONALS

95. PRINTED MENU for the 'Dinner of the Society of Anaesthetists at Limmer's Hotel 15th October, 1896'. (WLMS 5461/71)

CASE 6: ANAESTHESIA AND INNOVATION

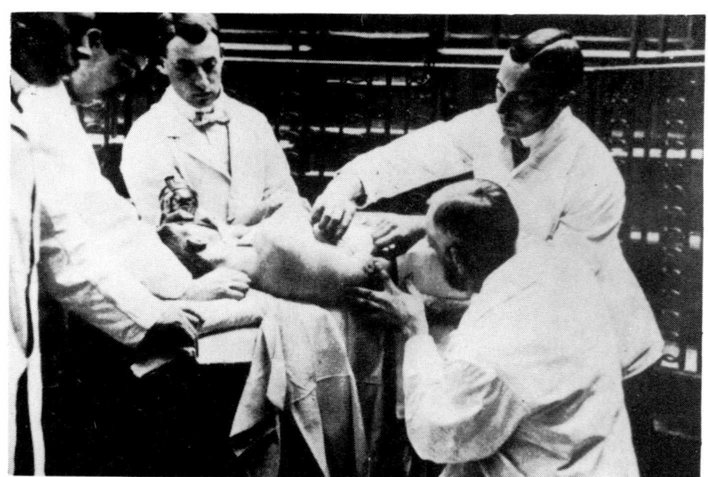

Item 101

Within a year of the introduction of ether anaesthesia to Britain, the *Pharmaceutical Journal* was able to publish reviews of numerous different methods of administration which had been described (see e.g. *Pharm. J.*, 'On the inhalation', 1846–7; ibid., 'Apparatus for the administration', 1846–7). These ranged from the simple square of gauze to the hookah-like, glass contraption advocated by Tracy of Bart's (see *Anaesthesia and the Victorians*). Some forms of inhaler were clearly based on equipment related to pharmacy or inhalation. Squire's apparatus was modelled on Nooth's glassware for the preparation of carbonated waters. Inhalers such as Maddox's and Smee's resemble respirators designed to be worn over the nose and mouth to protect the wearer from harmful matter in the inspired air. These were widely advertised during the mid and late nineteenth century (see e.g. Arnold and Sons, 1880: 327).

A pattern of eponymous diversity prevailed in British anaesthesia until after the turn of the century. Before about 1855, many new inhalers were described in the pharmaceutical trade journals. After this date, the columns of *The British Medical Journal* and *The Lancet* were preferred, perhaps reflecting a growing tendency among medical men to give, or at least supervise, anaesthetics rather than call in a druggist or instrument maker with ideas and apparatus of his own.

Early descriptions of inhalers stressed convenience in use and transportability. Skinner's mask, for example, could be folded "so that it may be carried in the pocket, hat or case" (Duncum, 1947: 248). Later innovations were increasingly advocated on the grounds of greater safety for the patient. In particular, methods of regulating the dose of anaesthetic given were devised, together with new ways of vaporizing the agents. The inhaler designed by F.E. Junker (1828–1901) in 1867 was novel in its use of the 'bubble-through' technique, whereby volatile liquids were vaporized by passing air through them. The method proved to have hazards, however, most notably the tendency to pump liquid anaesthetic into the patient's mouth if the tubing was wrongly connected or the bottle tilted too much. Since the latter was hooked on to the anaesthetist's waistcoat pocket, this was perhaps not an unlikely occurrence.

Despite other criticisms, including the fact that it did not leave the administrator a free hand, it has been suggested that Junker's was the inhaler most commonly used with chloroform in late nineteenth century Britain (Duncum, 1947: 266). Numerous modifications were quickly produced, all on the grounds of increased safety. Junker's inhaler continued to appear in manufacturers' catalogues, and to be described in textbooks until the 1950s (e.g. Evans, 1951: 102). A detailed study of its use in the context of its perceived advantages and drawbacks would perhaps provide valuable insights into previous anaesthetic practice. It is startling to find, for example, that when suggesting methods of anaesthesia suitable for general practice in 1905, one author considered this small glass bottle, with simple tubing, hand bellows and facemask, too cumbersome for the country doctor, who, he said, "cannot be expected to go his rounds with a Krohne Inhaler in his pocket" (Krohne were the original makers of Junker's inhaler). The same author mentioned a further disadvantage for the single handed practitioner: "in the struggling stage the apparatus may be in the administrator's way and hamper him, or may get smashed up" (Luke, 1905: 85–6).

Nineteenth century innovations in anaesthesia involved, of course, not only new inhalers but new routes of administration and new anaesthetic substances. Benjamin Ward Richardson (1828–96), advocated the local effects of ether in 1866 as Hardy had done for chloroform vapour in 1854 (Hardy, 1854). In Hardy's case therapeutic, as well as local anaesthetic, effects were claimed and Pernick's recent work reminds us that innovation in anaesthesia should perhaps be considered in the wider context of medicine for pain relief (Pernick, 1985).

Rectal, regional and spinal anaesthesia had all been attempted by 1900, in Russia, Germany and the United States respectively (but see Proskauer, 1947, for a prior French claim). Spinal and regional anaesthesia utilized Carl Koller's (1857–1944) demonstration of the local anaesthetic properties of cocaine in 1884. The continued advocacy of techniques such as local freezing, however, despite their acknowledged inefficiency, is indicative of the frightening reputation that cocaine rapidly acquired for its unpredictable and sometimes fatal effects on heart and respiration, if allowed to enter the general circulation. Buxton considered that a dose of only half a grain "will in many people give rise to trouble" (Buxton, 1888: 134). Probyn-Williams restricted the total dose to less than $\frac{1}{2} - \frac{3}{4}$ grain. In his estimation, the British used local anaesthesia far less than their Continental or North American colleagues, preferring nitrous oxide for comparable procedures (Probyn-Williams, 1901: 195, 191).

Much early work on anaesthetic techniques remains relatively unexplored. Historians of anaesthesia often cite C.L. Schleich (1859–1922) as the originator of infiltrational anaesthesia by the injection of local anaesthetic drugs into the tissues. Schleich did use extremely weak solutions of cocaine and other drugs, but was primarily investigating the use of the physical effects of oedematization of tissues with a saline solution (0.2%) at lower than body temperature. "This was the essential condition required for the production of local anaesthesia. The small quantity of the analgesic drug that [Schleich] adds to his solutions is simply intended, he claims, to suppress the abnormal hyperesthesia of pathologic tissues" (Allen, 1918: 162).

Following the introduction of ether and chloroform, numerous other substances regularly stocked or easily prepared by pharmacists were investigated empirically for anaesthetic properties. Of these, bichloride of methylene enjoyed a certain popularity in Britain from the late 1860s until the 1890s (Sykes, 1982: 153–67). Richard Rendle (1811–93) of Guy's Hospital first used this agent in 1869. Having devised an inhaler, he later adapted it to another innovation, the use of anaesthetic mixtures. The 'ACE' mixture (absolute alcohol, chloroform, ether in a ratio of 1:2:3 parts), was popular from the time of its introduction in the 1880s until well into the twentieth century, though by then the alcohol was often omitted. In this form, one anaesthetist considered the mixture "a golden mean in the choice of an anaesthetic in all cases of doubt as to the most suitable" (Gardner, 1916: 160). As a means of reducing the total dose of any one agent administered, the principle was to find widespread application in twentieth century techniques.

Late Victorian Britain formed a particularly fertile field for the incorporation of the modifications and suggestions of those who administered anaesthetics into practical apparatus. A well-established manufacturing economy included a thriving pharmaceutical and surgical instrument-making trade which retained, and relied on, close contact with medical men in the design of new products. Comprehensive catalogues and well organised exhibitions, such as those which accompanied annual British Medical Association meetings, were an established feature of British commercial life (see e.g. *BMJ*, 1868; ibid., 1888). This has been contrasted with the American situation, where anaesthetic 'gadgetry' never ousted the simple ether cone from pride of place in the early years.

In the twentieth century, the focus for anaesthetic innovation was largely industrial. In the fields of synthetic pharmaceuticals and precision engineering, the Germans and the Americans, respectively, were initially to take the lead (see *Anaesthesia and Industry*).

96. PHOTOGRAPH of Arnold and Sons, *A catalogue of surgical instruments*, London, Arnold and Sons, 1880, pp. 216–9.

97. CATALOGUE Arnold and Sons, *A catalogue of surgical instruments*, London, Arnold and Sons, 1880.

98. PHOTOGRAPH of the entry 'Anaesthetics' in the *Index-Catalogue of the Library of the Surgeon-General's Office*, Washington, Government Printing Office, 1880, vol. 1. p. 286. An indication of the vast number of publications on anaesthetic innovations.

99. RENDLE'S inhaler
1867–1920
A rounded, leather cone with air-holes at the apex and a flannel lining.
Richard Rendle (1811–93) invented this inhaler for bichloride of methylene in 1867, after experimenting with cardboard cylinders (Duncum, 1947: 264; Rendle, 1869). He introduced the new anaesthetic agent to the Eye Department of Guy's Hospital, London, where it was first given "like chloroform", then using cardboard cylinders lined with flannel. By 1870 it was used "almost exclusively" in that Department, "no accidents of any kind having yet occurred" (Bader, 1870: 100). The inhaler was subsequently adapted for use with ether, and ACE mixtures (alcohol, chloroform, ether, 1:2:3) in "Rendle's compendium sets". Rendle's inhaler was advertised until about 1915, but was increasingly criticised for uncertainty in dosage, freezing of the sponge and difficulty in cleaning (Blomfield, 1922: 115). F.W. Hewitt used a Rendle's inhaler during the operation on Edward VII in 1902 (Thomas, 1975: 44).
165 x 125 x 85 mm. A625372

100. GOLDAN'S Ether/Chloroform Apparatus
1880–1920
An anaesthesia kit comprising rubber facemask, two domed wire cages (one with gauze and lint padding), two metal tubes of differing lengths, each with five air holes at one end, and a rubber bag (missing from this example).
From these simple components a chloroform or an ether inhaler was assembled. For chloroform the facemask, shorter tube and wire cage with gauze were used. The more complex ether inhaler used the facemask, the shorter tube slotted into the longer so that the air holes could be open or closed, and the gauze-covered wire cage, covered by the rubber bag. This information is derived from three picture postcards, showing the inhalers when assembled, which accompany this example. They were produced by Reiger, 555, Third Ave., New York, and are annotated and signed S.O. Goldan – presumably the same Goldan who is known to have worked on spinal anaesthesia c. 1900 (Gwathmey 1914: 567).
longer tube 140 x 50 mm.
facemask 90 x 80 mm. A625443

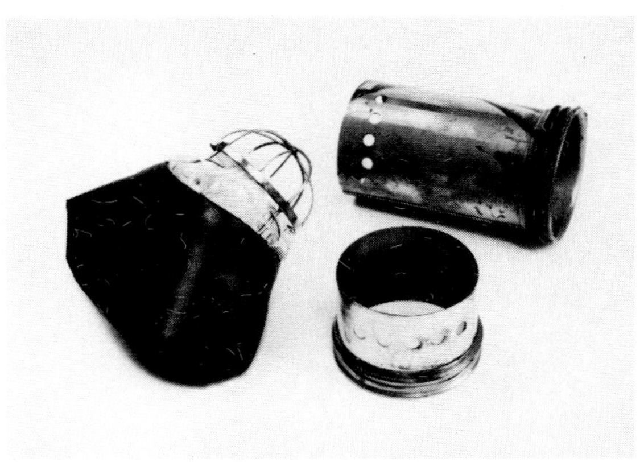

101. PHOTOGRAPH of the surgeon Rickman Godlee (1849–1925) operating at University College Hospital, 1899. The anaesthetist is using a Clover's portable ether inhaler or a modification. (From an original in University College Hospital)

102. PHOTOGRAPH of the beginning of an amputation at the Royal Infirmary Edinburgh, c. 1900. (From an original in the Royal Infirmary, Edinburgh)

103. JUNKER'S Inhaler
1867–80 *KROHNE & SESEMAN,/8, DUKE STREET, MANCHESTER SQUARE, LONDON, W.*
The inhaler comprises a screw-topped glass bottle encased in leather, with a scale of 1–8 painted on the leather adjacent to a vertical window allowing sight of the anaesthetic level. The cap incorporates a lapel hook. The cap also has mounts for afferent and efferent rubber tubing, the former extending as a metal tube almost to the base of the bottle, the latter ending immediately below the cap. Hand bellows, facemask and tubing are missing from this example. Described for use with bichloride of methylene in 1867 (Junker, 1867), this inhaler by F.E. Junker (1828–1901) was soon used for chloroform, and descriptions of its use recurred in textbooks until the 1950s (e.g. Evans, 1951: 102–3). Originally considered to deliver a known percentage of chloroform by a simple, 'bubble-through' technique, the inhaler underwent numerous modifications.
140 x 28 mm.
Loaned by The Pharmaceutical Society.

104. METHYLENE
1882–98 *J. ROBBINS & C0./147, OXFORD STREET, LONDON.*
Unopened bottle of methylene for anaesthesia in original blue paper packing. B.W. Richardson (1828–96) apparently introduced methylene into anaesthetic practice in 1867 (*BMJ*, 1867, 'Dr. Richardson'), although there has been debate as to the chemical nature of the substance he called bichloride of methylene (Sykes, 1982: 165–7). The anaesthetic had its devotees, including the ovariotomist, T. Spencer Wells (1818–97) (Wells, 1888). In 1888, Buxton described its use as "fraught with dangers" (Buxton, 1888: 103). By 1901, Hewitt considered that the "comparatively superficial" anaesthesia it produced "would hardly satisfy most surgeons of the present day" (Hewitt, 1901: 400).
110 x 40 mm.
Loaned by The Pharmaceutical Society.

105. HEWITT-JUNKER apparatus
1901–1936 *KROHNE & Co.*
A Junker's bottle, with etched scale *1–8 DRMS*, modified by the use of wide bore afferent rubber tubing to enclose the efferent tubing, which emerged from the former at right angles just above the hand bellows. Bellows, efferent tubing and facepiece are missing from this example. A chained stopper incorporating a filling funnel and a chained lapel hook are provided.
F.W. Hewitt's modification (Hewitt, 1901: 316–7) was designed to prevent confusion between afferent and efferent connections which, in Junker's design, had resulted in liquid chloroform being pumped into the patient's mouth. This example belonged to R.J. Probyn-Williams (1866–1952), author of an anaesthetic text (Probyn-Williams, 1901).
130 x 43 mm. 1983-881/94

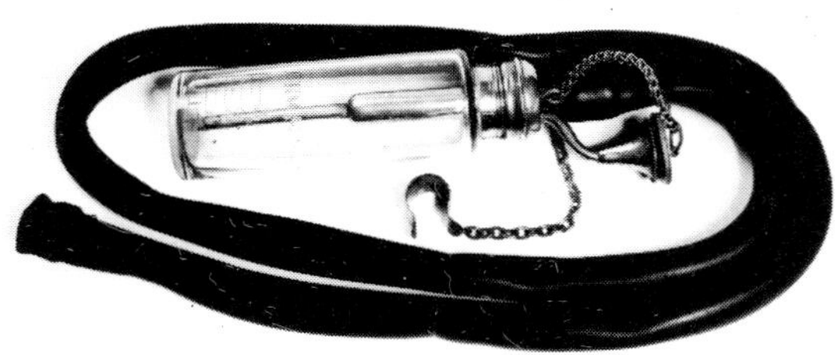

106. BUXTON'S IMPROVED Chloroform Bottle
1890–1930
A Junker's bottle, with etched scale *2–16 DRMS*, the metal mount having a trumpet-shaped filler cap and the internal, afferent tube protruding well below the shorter efferent within the bottle. A ceramic end piece is fitted to the afferent tube, to prevent freezing and blocking of the tube (see Buxton, 1914: 256).
The bottle from Buxton's Improved Junker Apparatus, introduced c. 1890, was incorporated into other modifications, including Hewitt's. Buxton also designed a foot bellows in place of the hand-pumped rubber bulb (Buxton, 1888: 76–8; Idem., 1914: 256).
165 x 47 mm. 1983–881/141

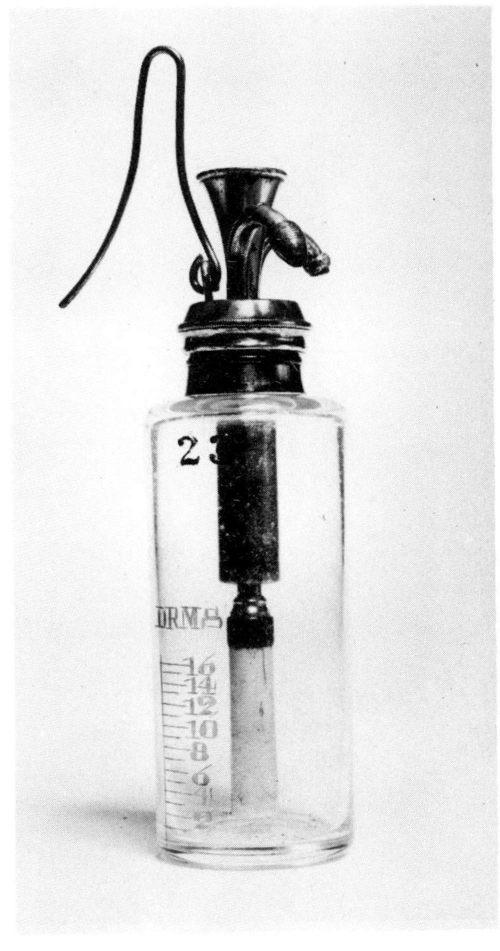

107. CARTER BRAINE'S Modification of Junker's Inhaler
1892–1930
A Junker's bottle of modified, 'hour-glass' shape. The longer, afferent tube is fitted with a flange to prevent liquid chloroform splashing into the short efferent tube.
A modification described by C. Carter Braine (1859–1937), anaesthetist to Charing Cross Hospital, London (Braine, 1892), this again incorporated features to prevent confusion between the afferent and efferent connections. They were given different outlet couplings. The bulbous bottle design was an extra precaution to prevent liquid chloroform entering the efferent tube, even when the bottle tilted. This example, probably Carter Braine's own, is connected to a flannel-covered mask.
220 x 110 mm. A625397

108. BRAUN Ether/Chloroform Inhaler
1901–40 *Narco*
Two rectangular Junker bottles, with moulded scales
for chloroform to *50 ccm*, and ether to *150 ccm*, in a
chromium-plated frame with communal metal mounts
for single dip tubes to each bottle, connectors for afferent and efferent rubber tubing and taps to control
the amount of air and vapour passing through the
ether and/or chloroform. A conical, plated metal,
valveless facemask with two air apertures, a leather
carrying thong, a right-angled mouth tube and a
wooden case are provided. Hand bellows are missing from this example.
J.T. Gwathmey (1863–1944) described this modification of Junker's inhaler as preferable to the Vernon
Harcourt inhaler (see *Anaesthesia and the Chloroform Question*) (Gwathmey, 1914: 323). It could be
used for ether or chloroform or mixtures of the two.
The inhaler was devised by H. Braun (1862–1934) of
Göttingen in 1901, an account appearing in the *BMJ*
that year (*BMJ*, 1901: 96; Thomas, 1975: 219–24).
This example was owned and used by a Dr. J.D. Whit-
ney of London, from about 1910–1940.
case 107 x 235 x 215 mm. A500269

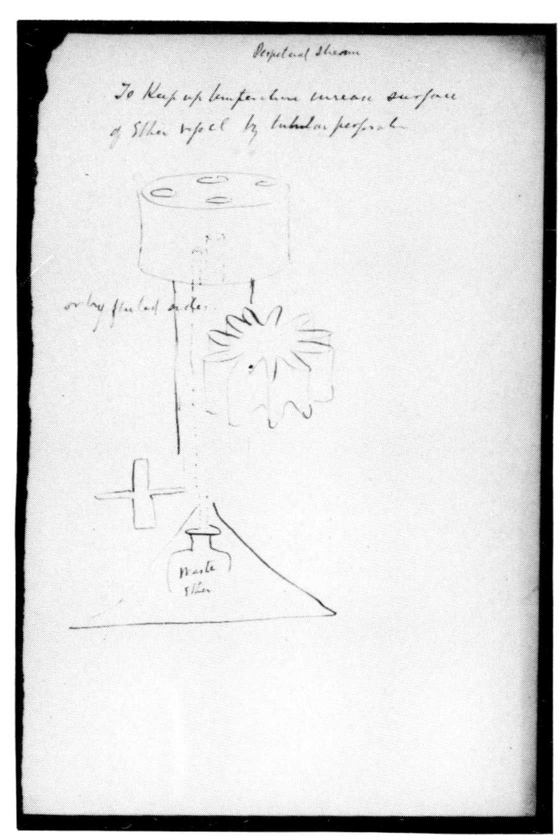

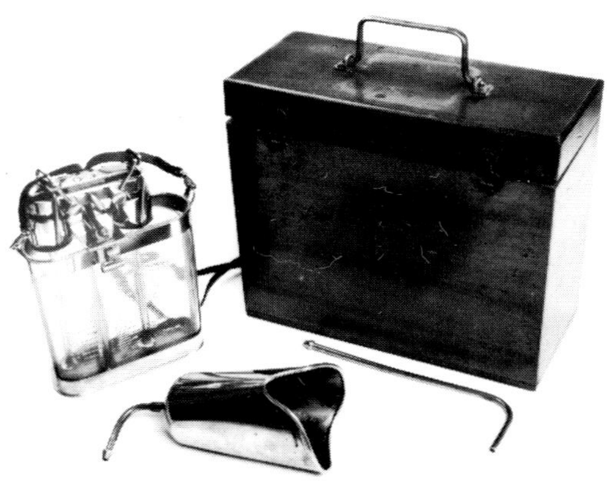

JOSEPH T. CLOVER (1825–82)

109. HAND-BILL advertising 'Clover's portable regulating ether inhaler', by Mayer and Meltzer, 71,
Portland St. [London], c. 1877. "£3" – hand written
on upper left corner (Moorat 1973: MS 1685).

110. DRAWINGS A selection of manuscripts with
drawings of anaesthetic apparatus by J.T. Clover.
Clover seems to have been an inveterate scribbler and
designer, drawing on any odd piece of paper. c. 1870
(Moorat, 1973: MS 1684).

111. HAND-BILL advertising 'Clover's gas and
aether inhaler', by Mayer and Meltzer c. 1876. Hand
written, "Inhaler and bottle of gas £11.0.0., with 2
bottles £14.0.0." (Moorat, 1973: MS 1685).

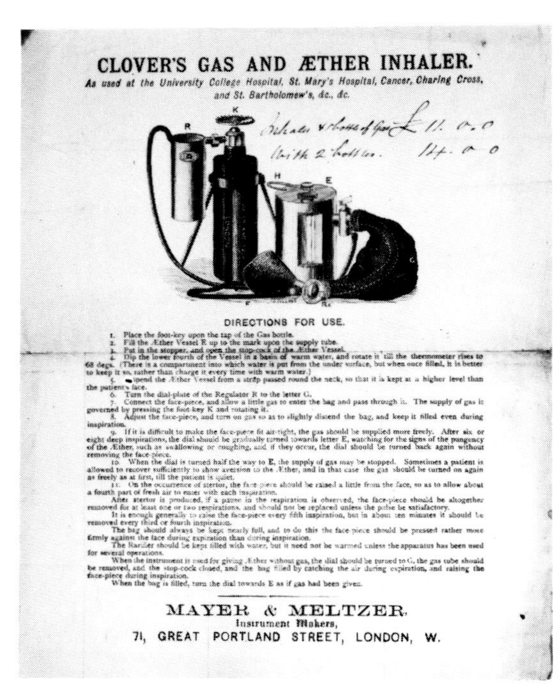

INTRAVENOUS ANAESTHESIA

112. CHLORAL V. Deneffe and A. Van Wetter, *Nouvelles études sur l'anesthésie par injection intra-veineuse de chloral*, (Reprinted from *Bull. Acad. roy. Méd. Belgique*, 3 ser. *10* (6)) Brussels, Henri Manceaux, 1876.

LOCAL ANAESTHESIA

113. RICHARDSON'S SPRAYS for local ether
1866–1910 *ARNOLD & SONS/LONDON*
Mahogany case containing a round, clear glass bottle, with two etched scales, 1–32 drachms and $\frac{1}{2}$–4 fluid oz., and ground glass stopper with chamois leather cover and printed label: Methylated Ether. W. Martindale, Pharmaceutical Chemist, 10 New Cavendish St., Portland Place, London W. A second glass bottle with moulded scale *0–12 DRS* is included. A metal spray attachment, inserted through a cork, fits the first bottle, and a vulcanite attachment, with two alternative nozzles, fits the second.
Benjamin Ward Richardson introduced an ether spray for local refrigeration anaesthesia in 1866 (Richardson, 1866). Buxton described it as an alternative to the injection of cocaine – which was used with great trepidation – but found its anaesthetic effect "very transient", recovery of sensation "very painful" and "the use of the knife almost impossible" owing to a thick coating of ice on the skin and instruments. Sloughing, "like that of frost-bite" was a further complication (Buxton, 1888: 143). Richardson's use of the hand bellows that worked this type of spray (missing from this example) was subsequently followed in, among other devices, the Lister carbolic spray (see Duncum, 1947: 29–30).
bottles 110 x 56 mm. and 85 x 46 mm. 1983–881/134

114. COCAINE POTS
1890–1930 *MAYER & CO/LONDON*
Two plated metal pots, with weighted bases and stand, donated to the Royal College of Surgeons of England by Charles Heath (1856–1934), an ear, nose and throat surgeon. Similar glass pots, described as "Chas. Heath's pattern" appear in Mayer and Meltzer's catalogue of about 1914 for hypodermic cocaine (Mayer and Meltzer, c. 1914: 340). The endoscopist, Chevalier Jackson (1865–1958) described similar porcelain containers for cocaine solutions of two strengths, in which tampons for packing into the larynx were soaked (Jackson, 1923: 40, 59).
pots 30 x 25 mm. 1983–881/388

115. CHLOROFORM S.L. Hardy, *A practical inquiry on the vapour of chloroform as a local application*, Dublin, Thomas Deey, 1854. Presented by the author to the physician John O'Brien Milner Barry (1815–81), with autograph presentation letter inserted, dated Dublin May 14, 1855.

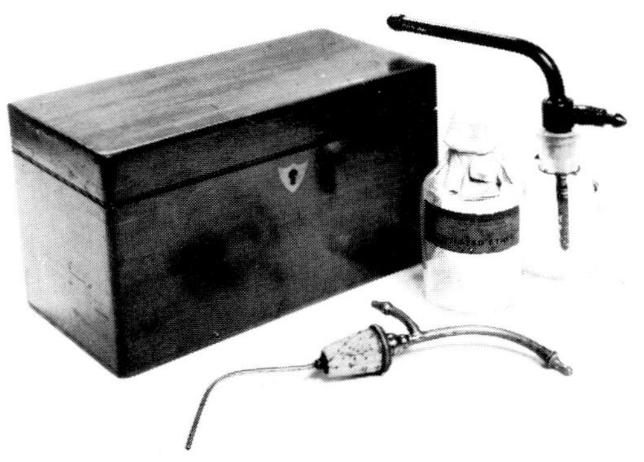

CASE 7: ANAESTHESIA AND TECHNICAL SOLUTIONS

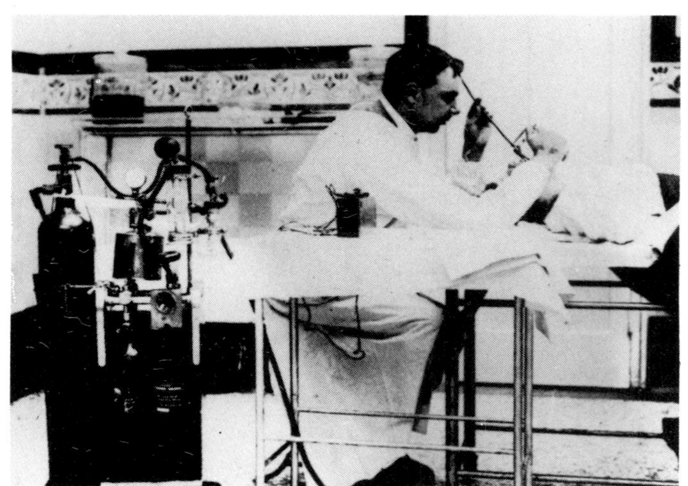

Item 118

The history of anaesthesia has often been written as though it were a series of solutions to technical difficulties confronting surgeons. This is hardly surprising. The successful deployment of complex anaesthetic apparatus in operations and situations inconceivable fifty years ago seems an obvious end point for a history. This approach, however, avoids the wider question of why certain issues were identified as technical problems within the surgical or anaesthetic realm and not defined in other ways. Current ethical dilemmas, such as the use of respirators to prolong life in brain damaged people, are not simply a modern problem suddenly produced by new technology. They are the outcome of an historical process in which, at various stages, 'problems' were defined as technical rather than for example, social or moral (for an alternative historiographical model see Pinch and Bijker, 1985).

In a number of contexts, anaesthesia entered nineteenth century medicine as a technical adjunct to problems already conceived of as surgical, rather than being used to redefine the domain of surgery. For example, in 1864 James Syme (1799–1870) performed a massive resection of the tongue and jaw without an anaesthetic because its use would have interfered with his work (Syme, 1865). From the very early days access to the mouth challenged the ingenuity of anaesthetic innovators (Sykes, 1982: 92–112). The problems posed by oral surgery were competition for space between the surgeon and the anaesthetist, and the danger of the unconscious patient inhaling blood. The latter difficulty was usually overcome by using light anaesthesia and allowing the patient to cough. Indeed "Reflex movements and vocal sounds were ... the rule" in all anaesthesia for, perhaps, twenty years after 1846 (Hewitt, 1901: 19). The problem of access was usually addressed by modifying the anaesthetic apparatus employed or by using gags and tongue depressors. Preliminary tracheotomy was also tried. Technical difficulties and different perceptions of pain, however, ensured that tonsillectomy was sometimes performed without anaesthetic by general practitioners in Britain, until the interwar years.

Another solution to these and other problems was 'intubation', passing a tube through the mouth or nose into the trachea (Duncum, 1947: 597–613). The technical lineage of this now common method of administering anaesthetics is customarily traced to the invention of a practical intubation tube by Joseph O'Dwyer (1841–98) in 1885. The early use of intubation in anaesthesia was also closely related to clinical and experimental work on problems associated with thoracic surgery, notably maintaining a pressure sufficient to prevent collapse of the lung. There is an excellent technical history of this subject (Mushin and Rendell-Baker: 1953). These authors show that, during the first decade of this century, a range of positive and negative pressure machines was devised for use in anaesthesia and for the artificial respiration of paralysed patients. They were of course marginal to regular clinical practice.

A monograph could undoubtedly be written on the endotracheal catheters, tubes and laryngoscopes which were devised before 1940, in order to circumvent particular anaesthetic problems. However it is generally agreed that the work of Ivan Magill (1888–1986) and Edgar Rowbotham (1890–1976), published in 1921, was fundamental to the creation of modern anaesthetic practice. Magill and Rowbotham worked with soldiers who had sustained maxillo-facial injuries during the Great War. To produce satisfactory anaesthesia they used Shipway's warm ether apparatus and wide-bore endotracheal tubes (Rowbotham and Magill: 1921; see also Thomas 1975: 175–205). Magill also introduced a laryngoscope that was much favoured by British anaesthetists. The use of warm ether vapour had been reintroduced during the First World War (see *Anaesthesia and Two World Wars*). Ether at room temperature dropped on to a mask produced a marked fall in temperature, sometimes such that frost formed and further inhalation became impossible. Victorian doctors had suggested the use of warm ether to overcome this difficulty but a satisfactory device had not been produced. Francis E. Shipway (1875–1968), in 1916 Honorary Anaesthetist to Guy's Hospital, was one of those responsible for reintroducing warm ether which he gave with a device of his own design based on the Junker bottle (see *Anaesthesia and Innovation*) (Shipway, 'Advantages' 1916).

Between the start of the First War and the end of the Second, a great number of technical innovations were introduced into anaesthetic practice. These included the use of carbon dioxide absorbers to make the recycling of agents possible, an invention which had important economic corollaries. After the introduction of cyclopropane, anaesthetists in the 1930s began to use the gas to produce deep anaesthesia, paralysing the patient's own respiration and controlling the inflation of the lungs by rhythmically squeezing a rubber bag incorporated in the circuit. The introduction, in 1943, of curare as as an agent for inactivating the respiratory muscles, enabled anaesthetists to produce the same effect much more simply. By the end of the Second World War therefore, the fundamental technical practices of much modern anaesthesia – intubation, mechanical ventilation and muscle relaxation – had all been employed in one context or another. Most everyday anaesthesia at this time, of course, still used a facemask and the patient's own respiratory exertions. It was changes on a wider scale – in the practice of surgery, in the relationship of medicine to industry, and in the role of hospitals – which eventually established current anaesthetic practice.

GENERAL SURGERY

116. PHOTOGRAPH of the surgeon Sir John Bland-Sutton (1855–1936) with the anaesthetist R.E. Apperly (1883–1960), at the Middlesex Hospital, London, c. 1915. Not all anaesthetists welcomed technical innovations. Apperly, described as "a magician with a rag and bottle" was "very anti anything by injection" because as he said, once "it's in you can't get it out" (W.R. Winterton FRCOG, personal communication). (From an original in the Middlesex Hospital)

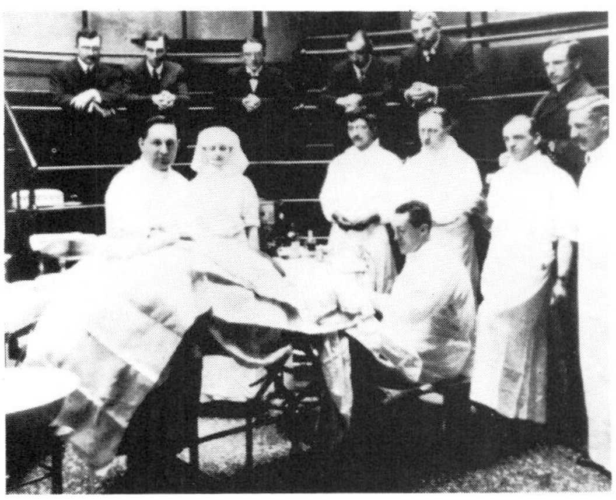

INTUBATION

117. PHOTOGRAPH of intubation, using a laryngoscope c. 1920.
(From an original in the possession of Dr. David Wilkinson)

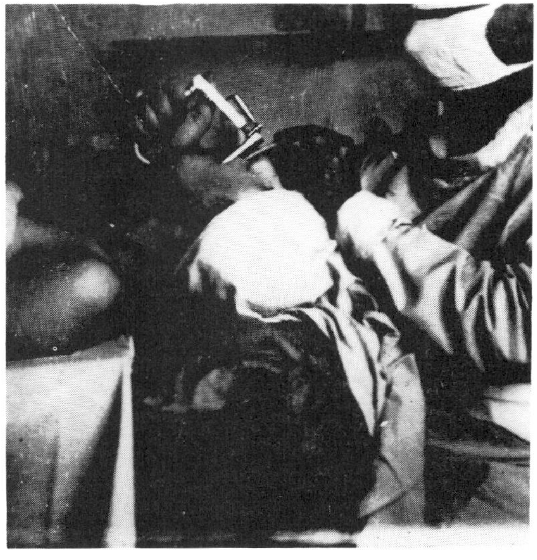

118. PHOTOGRAPH showing the anaesthetist passing a gum elastic catheter into the trachea, c. 1920. (From an original in the possession of Dr. David Wilkinson)

119. FELL-O'DWYER Apparatus.
1888–1910

A curved metal tube for insertion into the mouth and larynx, with a flanged external end, designed to be covered by the operator's thumb during inflation. The tube has a side-piece for the attachment of tubing from foot-operated air bellows. Three finger rings and four interchangeable conical heads (two of metal and two of vulcanite), to secure an airtight fit in the larynx, are provided. The set includes a smaller laryngeal tube and head for a child and is packed in a leather case.

E.G. Fell (1850–1918), ear, nose and throat surgeon of Buffalo, USA, applied a resuscitation technique well known in laboratory animal work to human subjects in 1887. Air from bellows was pumped into the lungs via a tracheotomy tube or facemask. Joseph O'Dwyer (1841–98), working on intubation of children with diptheria, adapted Fell's apparatus for use with his laryngeal tubes in about 1888. In 1899, Rudolf Matas (1860–1957), used the Fell-O'Dwyer apparatus to give an anaesthetic by adding a gauze-covered cone on to which liquid anaesthetic was dropped, to an extra sidetube (Mushin and Rendell-Baker, 1953: 44–5). These methods were certainly not part of most anaesthetists' experience. Intubation did not find a role in either routine practice or emergency resuscitation until much later. Writing in 1901, Hewitt describes inflation of the lungs as having fallen into disuse "at the present time it is rarely if ever employed" (Hewitt, 1901: 464).

case 250 x 103 x 36 mm. 983–881/326

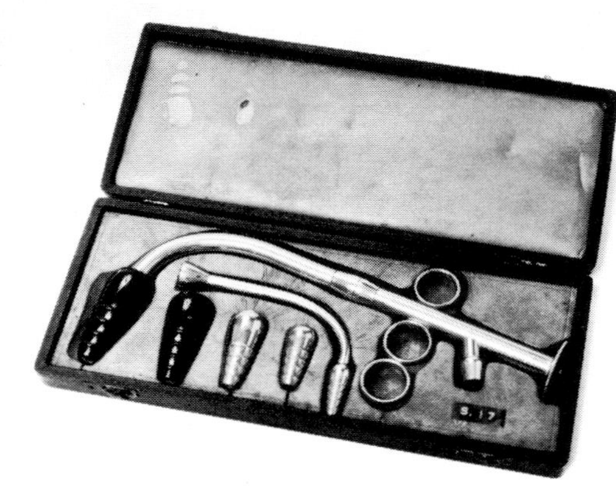

LARYNGOSCOPES

120. MAGILL laryngoscope
c. 1950 *A. CHARLES KING. LTD.*
210 x 135 mm.

121. MAGILL-GUEDEL laryngoscope
c. 1950 *A. CHARLES KING*
190 x 190 mm.

122. RAE-TYPE laryngoscope
c. 1950 *KING. LONDON*
190 x 180 mm.
Loaned by Dr. David Wilkinson, St. Bartholomew's Hospital.

TONSILLECTOMY

123. PHOTOGRAPH of a tonsillectomy operation at the Highgate New Town Clinic, London, c. 1925. (Copyright Greater London Photographic Library 80/5359)

124. MEDING'S enucleating snare for tonsillectomy
1920–1935 *DOWN BROs. LONDON*
300 x 72 x 19 mm. A612783

125. GUILLOTINE for tonsillectomy
1850–1900
180 x 22 x 94 mm. A612876

126. ELPHICK tonsillotome
1900–30 *ALLEN & HANBURYS/LONDON*
188 x 56 x 156 mm. A612877

MOUTH GAGS

127. FERGUSSON'S mouth gag
1900–35 *D.M.C. ENG* (The Dental Manufacturing Company)
192 x 109 x 54 mm. A613149

128. MASON'S-TYPE gag
1880–1900 *MAYER &/LONDON/MELTZER*
127 x 37 x 35 mm. A650752

129. DOYEN'S gag
1895–1930 *ALLEN & HANBURYS/LONDON*
130 x 85 mm. A56665

130. BOXWOOD SCREW gag
1880–1920
69 x 31 mm. A56726

ETHERIZATION

131. APPARATUS for warming anaesthetic
1900–30

Heavy-bottomed glass jar, containing a coiled copper tube and covered by a brass plate and fittings. The coiled tube connects at its base to an arched copper pipe with tap on the brass plate, and from its top to a short length of copper tube projecting above the plate. A central, screw-capped, funnel-shaped inlet in the plate connects to a straight copper tube leading almost to the bottom of the jar. A brass tap with a connection for rubber tubing enters directly into the glass chamber.

This apparatus is described as being for 'warming anaesthetic' in the descriptive catalogue revised for the Royal College of Surgeons of England by W.E. Thompson in 1952, it being one of the items donated

by N.St.J.G. Dudley Buxton in 1932 (Royal College of Surgeons, 1952: no. 19.57). Its method of use is unclear. Between about 1900 and 1930, several means of delivering warm ether vapour were devised which bear some resemblance to this apparatus. Most involved vaporizing the ether in a separate container and passing the vapour through a coil immersed in hot water (e.g. Sington's apparatus, Allen & Hanburys Ltd., 1930: 34; for a survey of warm ether methods to 1900, see Duncum, 1947: 582–90).
144 x 89 mm. 1983–881/148

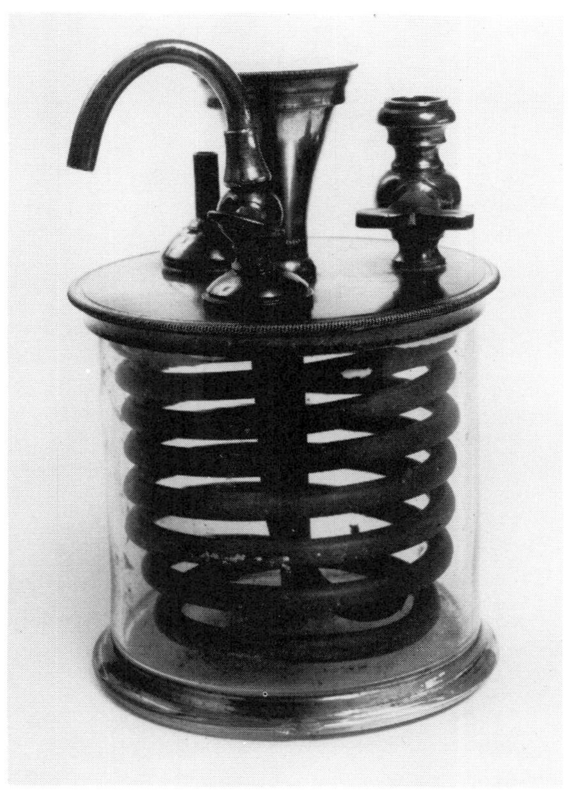

132. SHIPWAY'S Warm Ether/Chloroform Intratracheal Apparatus
c. 1940 *ALLEN & HANBURYS Ltd/LONDON*
A 'Junker' bottle for chloroform, an ether bottle and a vacuum flask, in a nickel-plated triple canister, which also acts as a water bath for the ether bottle. A metal U-tube passes into, and out of, the corked vacuum flask, which was filled with hot water, (120deg.F) during use. Rubber tubing is connected and regulating taps are provided such as to allow the pumping of air through ether or chloroform, or both, or neither, thence, via the U-tube in the vacuum flask, to the patient. A hand bellows is missing from this example, which is a modification of Shipway's original design of 1916. This did not include the second tap, marked *0–1–2–3*, which regulates the amount of air which bypasses both ether and chloroform (Shipway, 'Advantages', 1916).
277 x 177 mm. A625499

133. SHIPWAY'S Warm Ether/Chloroform Intratracheal Apparatus
1916–35 *MAYER/LONDON*
A copper water bath to hold a waisted chloroform bottle and vaporizing chamber for ether beneath an ether reservoir with dropping control. Air, with or without oxygen, was passed through the anaesthetic agents by means of a motorized pump or foot bellows. A later version of Shipway's apparatus which he developed because his earlier version (see above) had been considered "too cumbersome and unnecessarily expensive" (Shipway, 'Insufflation', 1916). Nevertheless, the earlier version is illustrated far more frequently in trade catalogues and textbooks. The intratracheal cannula in this example is a replica.
255 x 286 x 285 mm. A625543

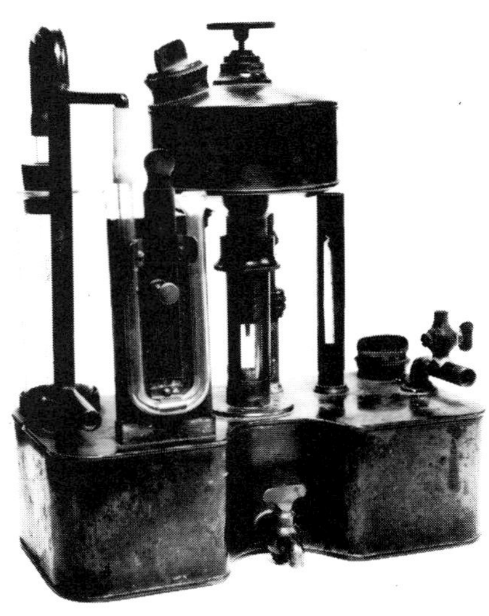

134. 'ELEKTRO PNEUMOSTAT' for etherization and suction
1920–40 *PAG*
An electric motor with rheostat control powers an air pump which is connected, via rubber tubing, to a facemask. The apparatus is encased in black plastic and fitted into a carrying case.
F. Kuhn (1866–1929), in 1905, was apparently the first to suggest removal of secretions from the respiratory tract by suction (Mushin and Rendell-Baker, 1953: 122). Electric motor-driven pump apparatus, which simultaneously administered anaesthetic vapours and removed blood and secretions from the field of operation, was advertised during the 1930s as especially useful for tonsil and adenoid operations (e.g. Down Bros, 1935: 1348). This example was supplied from the German manufacturer by Francis Riddell Ltd. of London.
case 317 x 312 x 128 mm. A625559

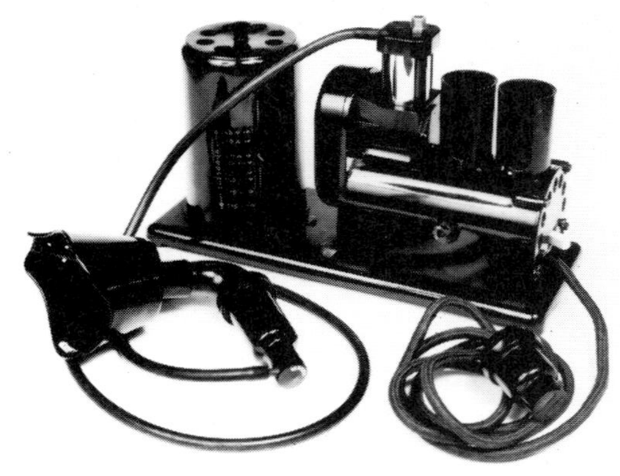

RECTAL ANAESTHESIA

135. BUXTON'S Apparatus for Ether Per Rectum
1906–32
A 500 ml clear glass jar to serve as a water bath for a 100 ml glass test tube for ether. Rubber tubing (now perished) connected the ether tube, via a glass intercepter (to prevent liquid ether entering the rectum) to the anal tube, which has a hooked, wooden handle, rubber cushion and bakelite rectal pipe. The intercepter is missing in this example.
Attempts, from 1847, to anaesthetize patients by the rectal introduction of liquid ether, or, later, ether vapour, met with mixed success. The *BMJ* in 1885 saw little future for the method, "though it may be useful for operations on the face or in the mouth"(*BMJ*, 1885, 'On anaesthesia'). D.W. Buxton (1855–1931) revived the practice specifically for this type of case, the method giving "greater facilities and freedom to the operator than any other plan" (Buxton, 1900: 137). He had added a special section on the method in oral surgery to this edition (the second) of his textbook. Evaporation of the ether was acheived by keeping the water bath at 120deg.F.
case 258 x 134 x 107 mm. 1983–881/330

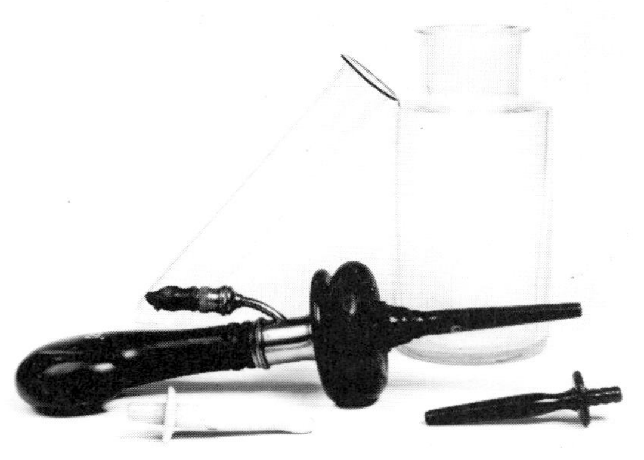

136. AVERTIN J. Kempson Maddox, *An introduction to "Avertin" rectal anaesthesia*, Sydney, Australia, Angus & Robertson Ltd., 1931. Showing 'Author's portable outfit for "Avertin" anaesthesia', f. p. 64. Avertin, Tri-brom-ethyl alcohol, was first used clinically in 1926. The authors recommended its employment in, for example, operations where cautery was in use about the head and an explosion therefore possible, and in "highly strung" patients.

CARDIAC SURGERY

137. RADIOLOGY Photograph of a patient being anaesthetised prior to angiocardiography (X-ray examination involving catheterization of the heart and injection of a radio-opaque dye), Sheffield. c. 1948 (*The British Journal of Radiology*, 1973, *43*: 745).

138. HYPOTHERMIA Robert W. Virtue, *Hypothermic anesthesia*, Springfield, Illinois, Charles C. Thomas, 1955. Local refrigeration anaesthesia was reintroduced in the early 1940s for amputation of atherosclerotic limbs. Hypothermic anaesthesia, the immersion of anaesthetised patients in iced water before operation, was introduced in the 1950s for operations on the heart and great vessels.

NEUROSURGERY

139. TRICHLORETHYLENE Philip Ayre 'Anaesthesia for neurosurgery with special reference to trichlorethylene', *British Journal of Anaesthesia*, 1944, *19*: 17–31. The author described an "open" method of giving nitrous oxide to carry the vapour of trichlorethylene. The object was to reduce brain or spinal cord haemorrhage said to be caused by raised intracranial pressure owing to the rebreathing bag employed in the "closed " method. Local anaesthesia was often the method of choice in neurosurgery, especially in America (Lazorthes, 1954).

VENTILATION

140. BEAVER Respirator, Mark II
c. 1960 *THE BRITISH OXYGEN COMPANY LIMITED/MEDICAL DIVISION LONDON and BRANCHES*
A small electric motor to expand and compress a rubber concertina reservoir bag from which air, or oxygen, is delivered to the patient. Operating instructions are given on a side panel (the internal construction of this type of ventilator is described by Mushin *et al.*, 1969: 313–20). Like many similar devices to inflate the lungs of paralysed patients, often manually, via a tracheotomy tube, this was introduced in the wake of the 1952 poliomyelitis epidemic in Copenhagen (Beaver, 1953). This model was portable, and this particular example was used in the wards of Darlington Memorial Hospital, the four hooks at the base of the housing being for carrying straps.
335 x 335 x 470 mm. A662288

CASE 8: ANAESTHESIA AND WOMEN

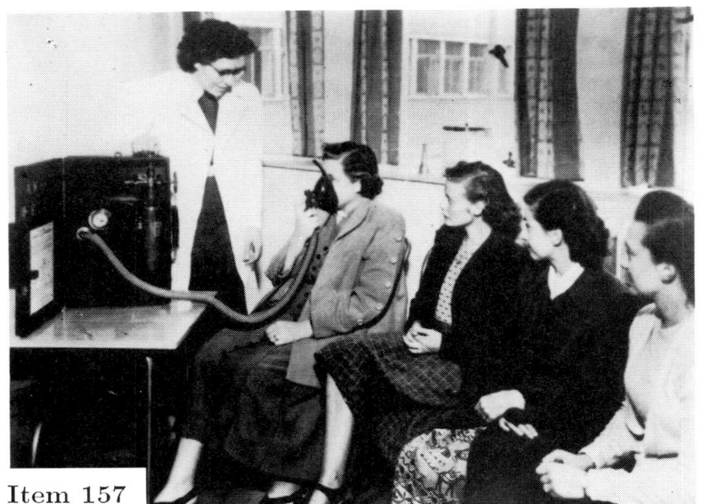

Item 157

The inclusion of a section entitled 'Anaesthesia and women' in this exhibition is intended to take into account recent work in the history of medicine and, since the 1960's, in wider cultural studies of all kinds. Earlier this century, analagous exhibition spaces might have been more narrowly entitled 'Anaesthesia in Childbirth'. Since then, a great deal of effort has been expended in some quarters in demonstrating wider privations and inequalities in the female role. According to these accounts, where women have come into contact with the predominantly male medical profession, the combination has been a recipe for exploitation. Obstetricians and gynaecologists have come in for particularly heavy criticism (see e.g. Oakley, 1984). We still lack, however, a substantial foundation in detailed historical studies of the origins of modern obstetric practice in general and of the management of pain in labour in particular.

For earlier historians of anaesthesia the introduction of effective pain relief in childbirth was represented as an episode in which enlightened rationality triumphed over religious bigotry (see e.g. Claye, 1939). More recent work, however, has suggested that opposition to anaesthesia in childbirth came, to a large extent, from other quarters. In the context of the various theories which underpinned mid-nineteenth century therapeutics, 'debilitating' women in labour by means of anaesthesia could have been perceived as an occasionally necessary evil or a contravention of basic principles. As Martin Pernick has recently shown, opposition in America came not only from religious fundamentalists, but from the influential homeopathy and hydrotherapy schools. Both rejected anaesthesia in labour as "interference with nature's beneficial punishments" (Pernick, 1985: 50–3).

Of women's reactions to pain-relief in childbirth we know very little. Most compilations of experiences have been made to advocate particular techniques. Those included in accounts of 'twilight sleep' produced in the early twentieth century are examples of this kind (e.g. Rion, 1915; Tracy and Boyd, 1917; but see Sandelowski, 1984, for a recent reappraisal). The works of Grantly Dick Read (1890–1959), proponent of 'natural childbirth' in the 1930s and 40s, include, perhaps not surprisingly, statements from patients who obtained significant benefit from his techniques (see e.g. Read, 1943: 222–41). Almost non-existent are accounts from women who regretted the total amnesia of *Dämmerschlaf* or for whom Dick Read's relaxation methods simply did not work. The failure to seek out admittedly elusive material of this sort has allowed more recent historians as much freedom in making judgements about the past as their predecessors. For feminist historians, the oblivion of 'twilight sleep' deprived women of their rightful experience of, and control over, a supremely feminine function, whereas Dick Read's methods heralded the beginning of a new era of independence and, literally, raised consciousness (but again see Sandelowski 1984: 97 on the 'colonialization' of the Natural Childbirth movement by 'drug advocates').

Both traditional and modern conclusions about the role of anaesthetics in childbirth might be modified by more in-depth study. Some recent works have helped fill this gap. It is becoming apparent, for example, that in Britain most women delivered without anaesthetics or analgesics until the 1950s. This was partly a function of the fact that by far the greater number gave birth at home with the aid of a midwife, and until 1936 (1946 in Scotland) no unsupervised midwife was allowed to give an anaesthetic agent or strong analgesic without involving a doctor (Oakley, 1984: 110). The saga of the conflict between midwives and the medical profession, stretching from the eighteenth century to the present, provides a further context against which obstetric anaesthesia must be viewed (see Donnison, 1977). In this, as in the wider issue of the increasing medical supervision of childbirth itself, control of technologies, including anaesthetic apparatus, has been a factor of continuing importance.

Financial considerations also had a bearing on analgesia in labour. In Britain, before free medical care became available through the National Health Service in 1948, mothers paid directly for anaesthetic drugs. Nitrous oxide from Minnitt's apparatus cost substantially more than chloroform. Even after Minnitt's apparatus was approved for use by midwives in England and Wales, provided they had received special training and were accompanied by another trained person, many midwives could not afford to purchase the necessary machine. In 1939, only 0.5% of midwife − supervised home confinements involved the use of analgesics (Lewis, 1980: 146).

No anaesthetic was the cheapest of all, but lack of availability may have been related to the fact that, in the nineteenth and early twentieth century, some doctors asserted that women of 'primitive peoples' and of the 'lower orders' suffered less in childbirth than their more refined and wealthy sisters (Pernick, 1985). In Britain, in the 1930s and 40s, pain relief in labour became an issue in the debate over the falling birthrate, when surveys amongst working women suggested that previous traumatic deliveries deterred them from further pregnancies (Oakley, 1984: 130–1).

Almost unavoidably, it seems, newly studied aspects of the relationship between women and anaesthesia continue to involve issues of power and control (see e.g. Thatcher, 1953, for an idiosyncratic account of the nurse-anaesthetist debate). Most recently, these have encompassed the status of women anaesthetists themselves, who have been portrayed as thwarted specialists, as in the case of Virginia Apgar (1909–74), unable to acquire senior posts in their original choice of department. In the United States, it has recently been suggested, such women were careful to structure the anaesthetic departments to which they were perhaps unwillingly directed, such that they, at least, became a protected female preserve.

CHLOROFORM

141. SHOP ROUND for Chloroform
1801–1910
Chloroform continued to be used in British obstetrics until at least the 1940s, forming a frequent addition to general practitioners' bags, but also to be found in hospital practice. Manufacturers stressed its "time tested, durable" qualities as an anesthetic agent and the high level of purity attained in its preparation (Duncan, Flockhart, 1946: 32).
230 x 89 mm. A632516

142. CHLOROFORM 'BRISETTES'
1938–42 *J.F. MACFARLAN & CO/EDINBURGH & LONDON*
Gauze-wrapped glass ampoules, each containing 20 minims of chloroform, designed to provide 5–10 minutes pain relief when crushed. An extensive investigation into analgesics suitable for administration by midwives, conducted by the British (later Royal) College of Obstetricians and Gynaecologists in

1936, came to the conclusion that "chloroform by any method should not be used by midwives acting alone ... This finding should not, however, be taken as prejudicing the use of chloroform by registered medical practitioners" (British College of Obstetricians and Gynaecologists, 1936: 23). Brisettes continued to retail at about three shillings a dozen during the 1940s (Duncan, Flockhart, 1946: 132). They were withdrawn some time before 1949 (Evans, 1951: 105).
ampoule 76 x 15 mm. A625472

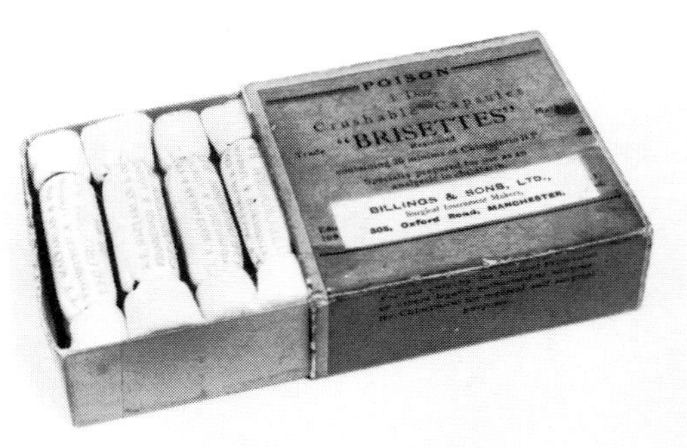

143. HOMEOPATHIC Medicine Chest
1850–1900
Wooden case containing forty-six glass phials (and
space for three more) of homeopathic medicines according to the system of Samuel Hahnemann (1755–
1843). Homeopathy achieved considerable popularity
in Europe and America in the late nineteenth century
and much opposition to pain relief in labour came
from its adherents. Like opium and morphine, anaesthetics were considered to interfere with beneficial,
'natural' pain (Pernick, 1985: 53–5).
70 x 70 x 36 mm. A656889

144. MURPHY'S Chloroform Inhaler
1850–1910
A simple metal box to hold a chloroform-soaked
sponge, soldered to a trumpet-shaped, silk-padded,
brass mouthpiece. Air entered through a variable
aperture in the lid of the box protected by a cloth
inspiratory valve. Expired air passed through a fixed
aperture, with a similar cloth expiratory valve, adjacent to the mouthpiece. An adjustable aperture connects the chamber to the mouthpiece. The nostrils
were held closed until the chloroform began to take
effect, then allowed to remain open. E.W. Murphy
(1802–77), Professor of Midwifery at University College Hospital, London, described his inhaler in 1848
(Thomas, 1975: 65). He was deliberately seeking pain
relief without loss of consciousness.
This particular example came from a cottage hospital
in Surrey. Murphy's inhaler continued to appear in
manufacturers' catalogues into the twentieth century.
In 1906 it cost 14s–6d, when Murray's mask (see below) cost 5s (Down Bros, 1906: 1078). The extent
of its popularity over more than fifty years is hard to
assess. Examples are frequently found in historical
collections (e.g. Thomas, 1975: 64).
115 x 76 x 54 mm. 1983–881/300

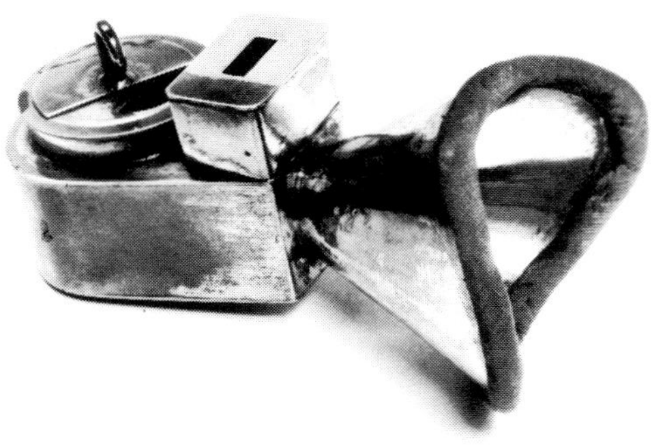

145. MURRAY'S MASK
1868–1900
A simple wire frame with flannel covering stitched
in place. John Murray (1843–73), chloroformist to
the Middlesex Hospital, introduced the design in 1868
(*Med. Times and Gaz.*, 1868).
120 x 77 x 65 mm. A600328

146. PROTHEROE SMITH'S Chloroform Inhaler
1847–57 *ARNOLD. MAKER*
A cylindrical glass vessel etched with the words
"Dr. Protheroe Smith's Inhaler" and scales from $\frac{1}{2}$–6
fluid oz. and 4–32 drachms.
The brass cover has two apertures, which were covered by screw caps when the inhaler was not in use.
One aperture connects with flexible, fabric-covered
tubing, the other is covered by a metal disc inspiratory valve, which may be adjusted by means of a
weighted lever. A wide glass tube descends beneath
the valve almost to the base of the container. Air
was thus drawn through the chloroform on inspiration. The mouthpiece, of painted metal, incorporates
two expiratory flap valves of leather. Protheroe Smith
(1809–89) claimed to be the first to use ether in obstetric cases in England, but soon followed J.Y. Simpson in using chloroform, for which he designed this
inhaler. He considered its greatest advantage to be
that it was "very portable" (Smith, 1847).
chamber 139 x 76 mm. 1983–881/150
mouthpiece 75 x 70 mm. 1983–881/331

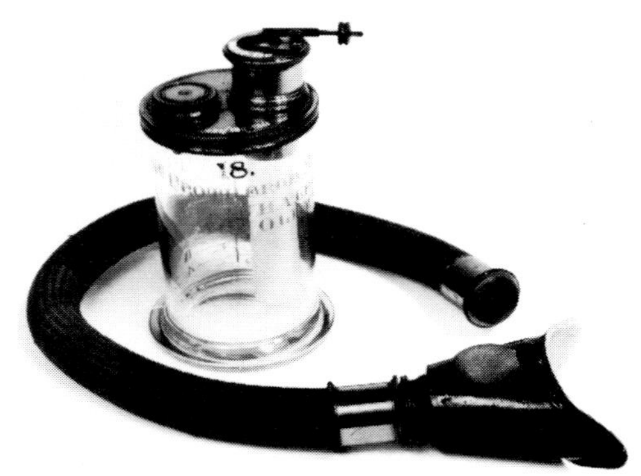

MIXED VAPOURS

147. VAPORIZING CHAMBER from Ellis's Inhaler
for Mixtures
c. 1870 *SAVIGNY & Co/67 St JAMES'S St.*
A cylindrical, compartmentalized, brass chamber engraved 'Mr. Robt. Ellis's Mixed Vapour Inhaler'. The
upper surface has two hinged aperture covers, labelled
alcohol and ether, and a central aperture, presumably
for the control drum, now missing, but described in
Ellis's May, 1866 version of his inhaler (Ellis, 'Additional note', 1866). This example differs in various
details from this version, also from that described
in June, 1866 (Ellis, 'Compound anaesthetics', 1866)
and from the example in the Charles King Collection (Thomas, 1975: 216). The internal structure includes, however, the metal frame supporting twenty
layers of cambric for the vaporization of alcohol which
Ellis described in May 1866 as an improvement on his
original design, which appeared in February that year
(Ellis, 'On anaesthesia', 1866).

Robert Ellis (1822–85) was obstetric surgeon to the Chelsea, Brompton and Belgrave Dispensary. His inhaler was developed in the context of increasing concern over the safety of chloroform, and the advantages claimed by the 1864 Chloroform Committee for anaesthetic mixtures, the 'depressant' chloroform being balanced by the 'stimulants', ether and alcohol (Ellis, 'Mixed vapours', 1866). Ellis recommended his inhaler, using all three agents, for anaesthesia in general surgery as well as obstetrics, the latter posing greater problems because of its 'prolonged' nature. He published no subsequent work on anaesthetics, "Not having the desire to win a reputation for giving anaesthetics only" (Ellis, 'Additional note', 1866) – an understandable sentiment in the 1860s, when specialization was still vehemently criticized by many in the profession. It seems his inhaler was not widely used. No entries have been traced in manufacturers' catalogues.

250 x 108 x 143 mm.   A625388

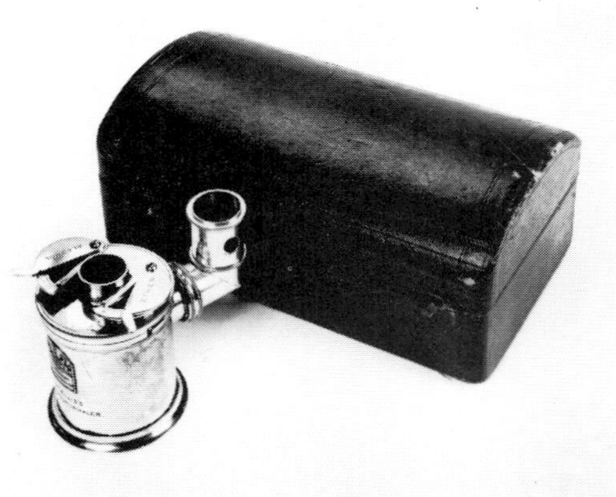

148. ANALGESIA Robert Ellis, *On the safe abolition of pain in labour and surgical operations by anaesthesia with mixed vapours*, London, Robert Hardwicke, 1866.

TRILENE

149. TECOTA MARK 6 Trilene Inhaler
1955–75 *CYPRANE LTD./KEIGHLEY/YORKS.*
A cylindrical, metal vaporizing chamber mounted on a reservoir for trilene resting on a base plate. A window to view the trilene level and a filler cap are provided for the reservoir, the internal construction of which resembles a 'non-spill' inkwell. Felt pads rise from this to the vaporizing chamber and the amount of air drawn through the chamber by the patient's respiration may be adjusted by the control dial above. A temperature-sensitive bimetal strip controls the size of the aperture conducting vapour to the patient, together with fresh air drawn through the apparatus.

A valve prevents rebreathing. The patient inhaled, through the rubber facemask and flexible tubing, at the beginning of each labour pain.

Following renewed interest in the anaesthetic properties of the volatile substance trichlorethylene ('trilene') during World War Two (see *Anaesthesia and a New Century*), several workers devised inhalers for its use in obstetrics, (e.g. Freedman, 1943). The concentration of vapour supplied from inhalers was found to vary substantially with temperature and with splashing of the trilene. H.G. Epstein (b. 1909) and R.R. Macintosh (b. 1897), working at Oxford University, devised the 'Emotril' inhaler (*E*pstein, *M*acintosh, *O*xford, *TRIL*ene) to solve this problem, in the hope of producing analgesic apparatus suitable for use by unsupervised midwives, who were then restricted in Britain to Minnitt's apparatus (see below). In some hands, Minnitt's apparatus had proved disappointing. "This may in some degree be attributable to the fact that the female is not mechanically minded" (Epstein and Macintosh, 1949: 1092). The Tecota Mark 6 worked on a similar principle to the Emotril. They were both finally approved by the Central Midwives Board for midwives' use in 1955 (Seward and Bryce-Smith, 1957: 42). This example came from University College Obstetric Hospital.

case 330 x 210 x 165 mm.   1984–1745

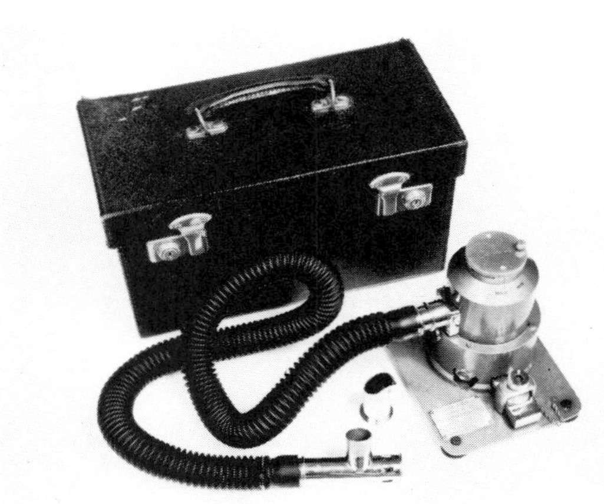

GAS AND AIR

150. WALTON-MINNITT Gas Air Apparatus
c. 1937 *COXETER/LONDON*
Wooden carrying case containing rubber facemask, tubing and a reducing valve, with spanner key for, and leather strap to support, a 100 gall. cylinder of nitrous oxide. A separate, glass-covered compartment contains a rubber reservoir bag beneath a hinged metal plate which is connected to the reducing valve of the cylinder. This is a portable apparatus designed for the self-administration, under supervision, of a fixed quantity of nitrous oxide gas mixed with air (approximately 45%). Nitrous oxide from the cylinder fills the rubber bag, which, as it expands, lifts

the metal plate to close off the supply of gas at the reducing valve. On inhalation the gas passes to the patient, together with air. R.J. Minnitt (1889–1974) designed his original apparatus, with the help of A. Charles King, in 1933 (Minnitt, 1943: 45). It was a modified form of an existing apparatus (McKesson's) for oxygen therapy. Minnitt's research was at the direct request of the Medical Board of the Liverpool Maternity Hospital, who were seeking an alternative to chloroform in obstetrics. The Board provided a research assistant and other facilities for assessing the new apparatus. By 1936, Minnitt was able to report on a series of 1,025 deliveries, and 400 examples of his apparatus were in use world-wide (Thomas, 1975: 237).

This particular model appeared in 1936, another followed that year (The Queen Charlotte), and in 1943 (The Standard) (Minnitt, 1944). Gas and air and analgesia from a recognized apparatus was approved for use by unsupervised midwives in Britain in 1936 (Minnitt, 1943: 46).

340 x 70 x 270 mm. 1981–986

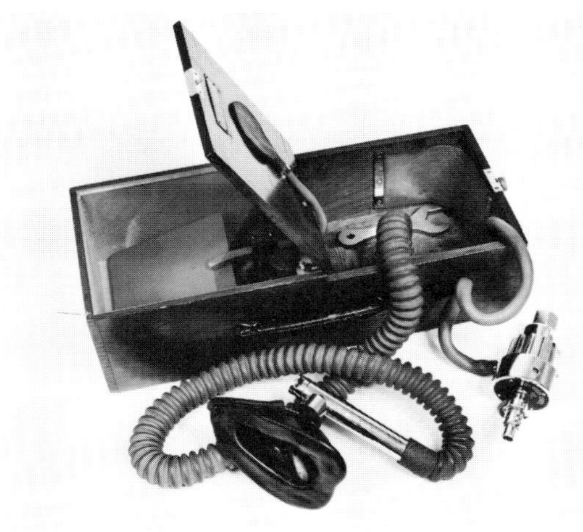

151. ANALGESIA R.J. Minnitt, *Gas and air analgesia*, London, Baillière, Tindall and Cox, 1938, signed "With Compliments A. Charles King" on the fly-leaf. Showing Fig. 9, 'Queen Charlotte's Gas-Air Analgesia Apparatus'.

152. PHOTOGRAPH showing administration of nitrous oxide and air from a Minnitt's apparatus during a home confinement attended by a London County Council midwife, 1949 (Greater London Photographic Library 26.82 F3561).

153. MIDWIFE'S HAT
c. 1950
Part of the uniform of a state certified midwife.
303 x 248 mm. 1982–561/35/10

154. INVESTIGATION British College of Obstetricians and Gynaecologists, *Investigation into the use of analgesics suitable for administration by midwives*, London, 1936.

155. ELIXIR British Schering Limited, *Oblivon in labour*, n.d. Advertising leaflet. Oblivon (Methylpentynol) was marketed in the 1950s, as an elixir to be given, with gas and air, to calm "nervous patients". (Loaned by Dr. David Wilkinson)

156. ANALGESIA Katherine G. Lloyd-Williams, *Anaesthesia and analgesia in labour*, London, Edward Arnold & Co., 1934, with a foreword by Dame Louise McIlroy. With the signature of A. Charles King on the fly-leaf and presented by him to the Royal Society of Medicine, 1940. (RSM)

157. PHOTOGRAPH Learning to use a gas and air machine, Woodberry Down Health Centre, 1953. (Copyright Greater London Photographic Library K1251)

THE NEWBORN

158. NEONATAL resuscitation outfit
c. 1955
Japanned metal case containing three oxygen cylinders by British Oxygen (with pencilled dates, 1956, 1958, 1965), reducing valve, rubber tubing and gas bag, green rubber facemask and mucus extractor. An emergency kit to deliver oxygen to the collapsed newborn infant via a facemask.

Greater attention was given to methods of neonatal resuscitation and ventilation after World War Two. General consensus on the usefulness of oxygen in this situation was reached by about 1950. Methods which did not involve intubation continued to be devised, much neonatal care being given by obstetricians and paediatricians, who were not necessarily skilled in intubation technique. During the 1960s, intubation came to be considered essential (Rupreht, 1985: 142–3).

case 340 x 70 x 270 mm. 1974–1746

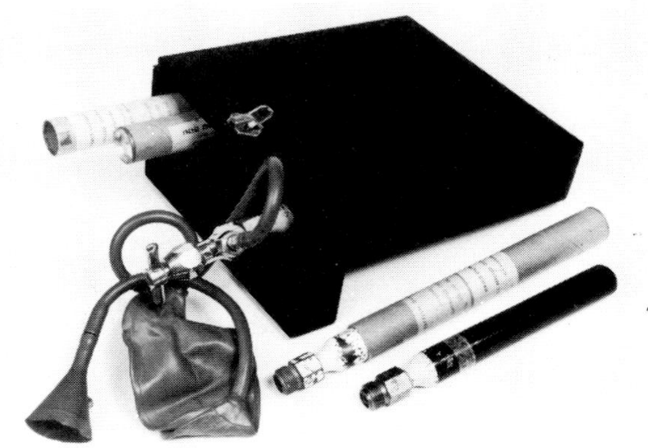

NATURAL CHILDBIRTH

159. MEDICAL OPPOSITION Grantly Dick Read, *Revelation of childbirth. The principles and practice of natural childbirth*, 2nd ed., 4th reprinting, London, William Heinemann, 1947.

160. PLATE showing ' "Sumner" the little son of Mrs Mark Boyd, born at Freiburg in January 1914', in Marguerite Tracy and Mary Boyd, *Painless childbirth. A general survey of all painless methods with special stress on "Twilight Sleep" and its extension to America*, London, William Heinemann, 1917, f. p. 191. 'Twilight sleep' was developed in Germany from 1902. It involved the use of injections of scopolamine (initially with a dose of narcotic analgesic). These caused mothers to forget any pain experienced, together with the actual events surrounding the delivery of their child. Several women from the United States travelled to Germany for their confinements following an article in *McClure's Magazine* in 1914 (Sandelowski, 1984: 3–26).

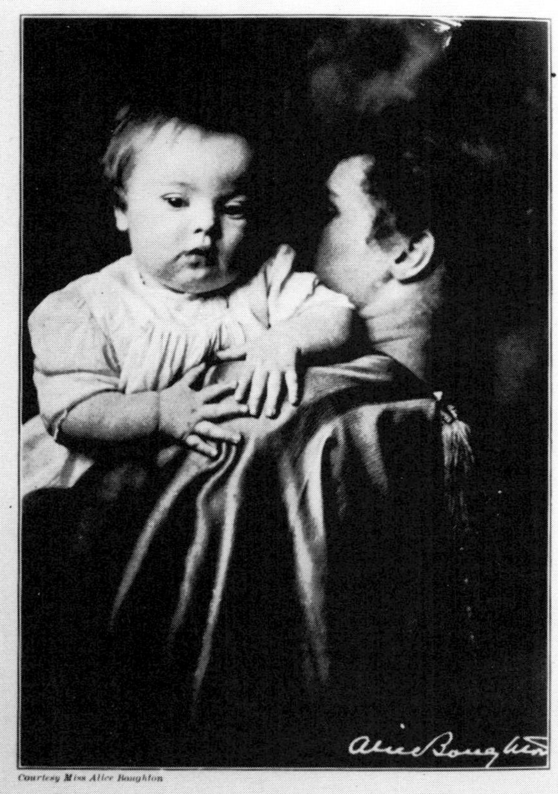

Courtesy Miss Alice Boughton

"SUMNER," the little son of Mrs. Mark Boyd, born at Freiburg in January, 1914. Mrs. Boyd turned an interrruption in the course of work into an opportunity for intensive work of a special kind.

161. PLATE entitled, 'A peasant mother and her twilight sleep boy', in Hanna Rion, *Painless childbirth in twilight sleep*, London, Werner Laurie Ltd., [1915], facing t. p.

162. SCOPOLAMINE William Osborne Greenwood, *Scopolamine-morphine semi-narcosis during labour*, London, Henry Frowde, 1918.

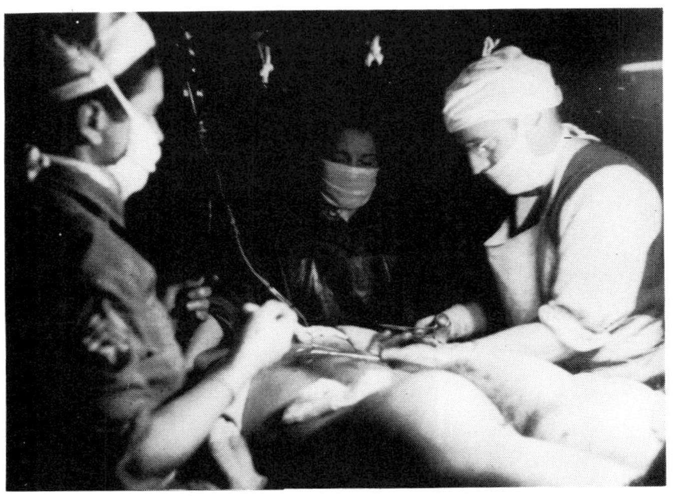

Item 170

The two World Wars were the theatres in which many innovations in anaesthetic technology were introduced. The conditions under which anaesthetics had to be given, the physical state of the troops and the peculiar nature of battle wounds all posed special problems in both World Wars. Many of the solutions to these problems became permanent features of anaesthetics in civilian life and many of them are well documented (Thomas, 1975). Rather less research has been done, however, on the organization of anaesthetic services in the wars, on the production, supply and transport of materials, and on the people who gave the anaesthetics. Chloroform had been the anaesthetic of choice in the Boer War. Because of its portability and the ease with which it could be administered it was widely used in general practice in Britain. Ether on the other hand, was favoured in America and in "surgical centres" in England (Hewitt, 1901:15). "At the commencement of hostilities chloroform was the only anaesthetic supplied at the front" (Macpherson, 1922: 178). In spite of its advantages, however, chloroform was found to produce post-operative deterioration in battle casualties and, except for the surgery of wounds of the chest, it fell out of favour.

Initially, in the British Army, anaesthetics were administered by the general medical officers but, in 1916, special anaesthetists were employed in the Casualty Clearing Stations. By 1918, there were also over 200 specially trained nursing sisters administering anaesthetics (Macpherson, 1922: 178). At the front a number of factors, not least the availability of materials, dictated which anaesthetic method was employed. Where possible, clinical considerations governed the choice of anaesthetic. For lightly wounded men and for amputations, gas and oxygen were recommended. Spinal anaesthesia was often found to be unsatisfactory because of its tendency to reduce the blood pressure in men who had been bleeding. Ether was usually the preferred agent. Initially it was given by the 'open method', that is by dropping it on to a mask. In men who had been living in trenches for six months, and who had numerous broncho-pulmonary complaints, open ether often produced respiratory complications. The 'closed method' was later adopted as it seemed to irritate the airways less. In the 'closed method' an inhaler, such as Clover's, with a bag is used. Even with this method a high proportion of soldiers with abdominal injuries died from pulmonary complications. This was said to be owing to pain, which restricted coughing and thus the expectoration of mucus or pus. Later, the apparatus designed by Francis Edward Shipway (1875–1968) (see *Anaesthesia and Technical Solutions*), in which warm ether was conveyed by an intratracheal catheter, began to be employed with success in these cases (Thomas, 1975: 182–5). This apparatus probably came into use in 1915, although its design did not appear in print until 1916 (Macpherson, 1922: 179). For operations on the head, local injection of novocaine and adrenaline were recommended, with the addition of systemic hyoscine and morphine if bone was to be cut (Marshall, 1917).

The First World War also saw the widespread employment of either atropine and morphine or 'Omnopon' – scopolamine as combined premedication (Gray, 1919) (see also *Anaesthesia and Women*). Shock was the condition which First World War anaesthetists recognized as their worst enemy. Although they could identify it clinically, they admitted that it was hard to define (Marshall,

1917). It was treated by warmth and fluid by mouth or per rectum. Intravenous saline was found to produce temporary improvement but no long term protection.

The Second World War saw a sharp decline in the number of deaths attributable to events associated with anaesthesia. A number of general and specific features contributed to this. First, the troops themselves were undoubtedly fitter than the men who had fought in the First War. Second, intravenous barbiturates, particularly pentothal, made it possible to avoid giving inhalational anaesthetics where they were contraindicated (see *Anaesthesia and Industry: One*). Intravenous drugs were also easily given by untrained personnel, although their excessive use at Pearl Harbor in shocked patients resulted in many deaths (Halford, 1943). Third, new agents such as vinyl ether and cyclopropane seemed to have definite advantages over ether in many circumstances. The most important factor in reducing the death rate, however, was the use of blood and plasma to combat shock. The ability to counteract shock also made spinal anaesthesia safer. This technique was extensively employed during the War, percaine being the drug most often employed in the British army. Boyle's apparatus, described in its original form during the First World War, which conveyed ether vapour in a gaseous vehicle, was widely used (Thomas, 1975: 145). A much more portable apparatus, the Oxford Ether Vaporizer, designed in 1941, was also extensively employed (Thomas 1975: 9).

Unlike the First World War, much of which was fought out in the trenches in France, the global scale of the Second War created special anaesthetic solutions to special problems faced by different branches of the forces. For example, in the Navy where equipment had to be "simple, strong, compact and easily replaced", the most basic equipment of all was often used: masks with drop bottles of ether or chloroform (Cope, 1953: 219).

In the long term, perhaps more important than the technical innovations it produced, the Second World War enabled anaesthetists to elevate their status and standardize their practice. At the beginning of the war only five regular officers in the British army had the diploma in anaesthetics (Cope, 1953: 220). Equipment was unstandardized and often inadequate. By the end of the war, standard, interchangeable parts were employed by a large number of skilled, specially trained anaesthetists. Early in the war Addenbrooke's Hospital, Cambridge, had advertised for nurses to undergo six months training as anaesthetists, a step which produced considerable controversy (*BJA*, 1941). British anaesthetists resisted dilution by what one of them called "the bane of the second rate American medical school, the nurse-anaesthetist" (Sykes, 1941).

WORLD WAR ONE

SURGERY

163. PHOTOGRAPH of an operating theatre at Wimereux, a village near Boulogne. World War One. Date and persons unknown. A sister is giving the anaesthetic.

164. GERMAN Military Anaesthesia Kit
c. 1915
A drawstring cotton bag, stencilled *Betäubungsgerät*, containing a folding, nickel-plated Schimmelbusch mask and two cotton covers with drawstrings. A nickel-plated funnel with removable filter is included in the set.
mask 190 x 110 x 40 mm. A655841

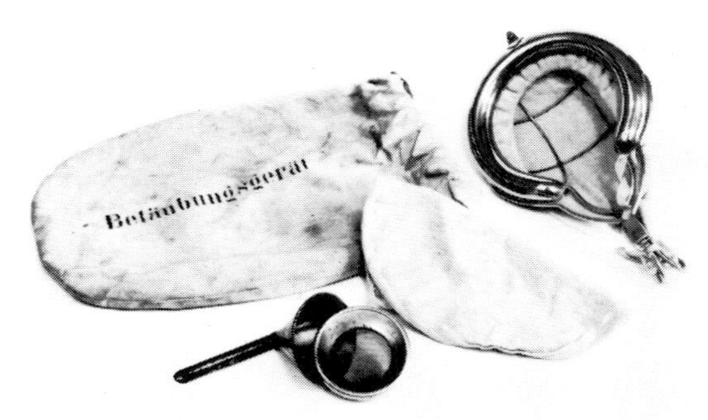

165. THE FRONT Geoffrey Marshall, 'The administration of anaesthetics at the Front', *The British Medical Journal*, 1917, i: 722–5.

PREMEDICATION

166. MORPHINE and Atropine for injection
c. 1924 *Burroughs Wellcome & Co.*
Morphine Sulphate gr. $\frac{1}{2}$ and Atropine Sulphate gr. $\frac{1}{100}$ for hypodermic injection. In twelve phials containing Wellcome tabloids to be dissolved in sterile water. A dummy pack for promotional or record purposes. The company first advertised the preparation in 1914.
57 x 47 x 17 mm. WFA EN/21

LOCAL ANAESTHESIA

167. PHOTOGRAPH of an advertisement by The Saccharin Corporation, Ltd., that one of its preparations, novocaine, a local anaesthetic, was unavailable "owing to the large requirements for the army and navy", *The Chemist and Druggist*, 1916, March 11: lx.

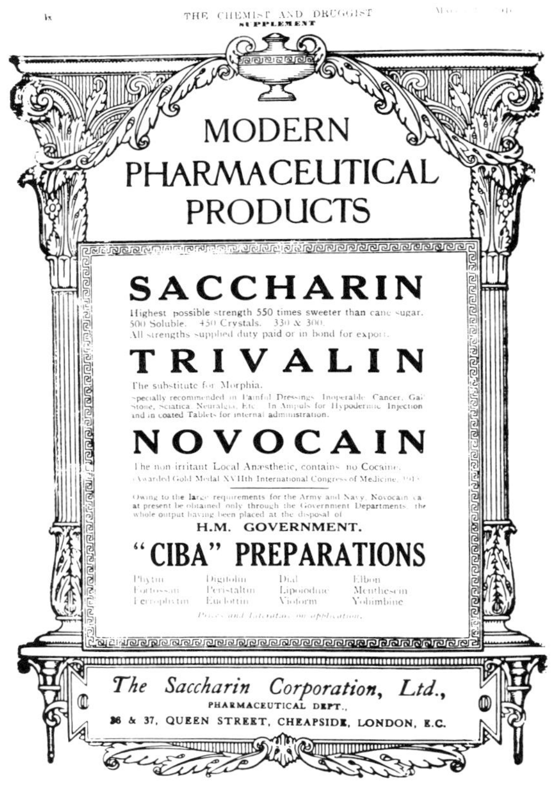

168. STOVAINE
1910–40 *PHARMACEUTICAL SPECIALITIES/ (MAY & BAKER)LTD. DAGENHAM.*
1 cc ampoule of stovaine (Amylocaine Hydrochloride), *Chaput formula* (10% stovaine, 10% sodium chloride, 80% distilled water).
Stovaine was synthesized in 1904, and was widely introduced for spinal anaesthesia as a less toxic substitute for cocaine. Stovaine was produced in two solutions, 'light' and 'heavy'. The latter, containing glucose, was supposed to act as a heavy foreign body and to move by gravity to the most dependent part of the dural sac around the spinal cord (Nosworthy, 1935: 173). Chaput's formula, which did not contain glucose, actually had a higher specific gravity (1.080) than the heavy solutions. Stovaine faced rivalry from novocaine (synthesised 1905) and by the late 1930s was regarded as unsafe (Evans, 1951: 251, 262).
40 x 10 mm. 1983–881/115

169. SPINALS May and Baker Ltd., *Stovaine* n.d. Promotional booklet. Stovaine was the spinal anaesthetic of choice in the British Army during World War One (Marshall, 1917). (Loaned by Dr. David Wilkinson)

WORLD WAR TWO

SURGERY

170. PHOTOGRAPH described as 'American and British Surgeons operating at 1st Division Casualty Clearing Station'. World War Two. Persons, place and date unknown (Copyright Trustees of the Imperial War Museum NA 11765).

171. 'E.S.O.' Chloroform Apparatus
1944 *THE LONGWORTH SCIENTIFIC/ INSTRUMENT Co. Ltd. OXFORD*
A khaki haversack containing a steel-cased anaesthetic apparatus in enamelled housing, comprising a vaporizing chamber for chloroform, hand-operated rubber 'concertina' bellows and flexible rubber tubing to facemask. A thermometer, graduated minus 20–plus 40deg.F, and a temperature dial are colour coded to allow for temperature compensation of the chloroform concentration (less air is drawn through the vapourizing chamber as the temperature of the liquid rises).
A certificate from the makers dated July 18, 1945, states that the apparatus, serial no. 63, "has been tested and approved and is issued complete with accessories and spare parts". The haversack is stencilled in ink: *M.E. Co. 1944* (the Mills Equipment Co., suppliers of webbing to the Army). The apparatus, the *Epstein – Suffolk – Oxford*, was produced by the

Nuffield Department of Anaesthetics, Oxford University, who were asked to design a dosimetric chloroform inhaler for parachute troops during World War Two (Epstein and Macintosh, 1949: 1092–3).
340 x 330 mm. A630946

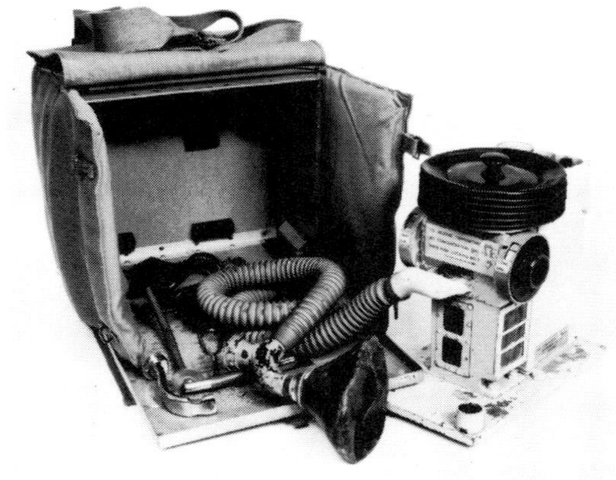

172. MILITARY Surgery Kit
1939 JETTER & SCHEERER/TUTTLINGEN
A steel case with carrying handles and removable instrument trays. A printed paper inventory inside the lid and an accompanying booklet enumerate the contents. These include, for anaesthetic purposes, a Schimmelbusch mask (now missing), dropping bottle stopper, airway and mouth gags. Spinal needles are also packed in the set.
515 x 310 x 160 mm. A619259

173. THE FRONT R. Blair Gould 'Anaesthesia for the badly wounded', *The Medical Press and Circular*, 1943, *210*: 151–3.

174. THE HOME FRONT F. Barnett Mallinson, 'Casualty surgery in the E.M.S.', *British Journal of Anaesthesia*, 1941, *17*: 98–107. E.M.S. was the Emergency Medical Service of the British Home Front. The author's favoured drugs were pentothal and cyclopropane.

ETHER

175. ETHER Can
c. 1930 E.R. SQUIBB & SONS/ NEW YORK.
Metal-capped canister containing 100g ether, with printed paper label, supplied in cardboard carton.
The cans in which ether was sold were adapted by Paluel Joseph Flagg (1886–1970) of New York for emergency anaesthesia and recommended for military use. The can was opened, emptied and refilled with the required amount of anaesthetic, air holes punched in the lid with scissors and a pharyngeal tube fixed over the central opening (Flagg, 1932: 148, 321). Thomas cites personal communications on the construction of similar emergency ether inhalers in the Spanish Civil War, 1938, and the Western Desert, 1940 (Thomas, 1975: 49–50). In the latter case, army ration cream tins were used.
86 x 53 mm. A625466

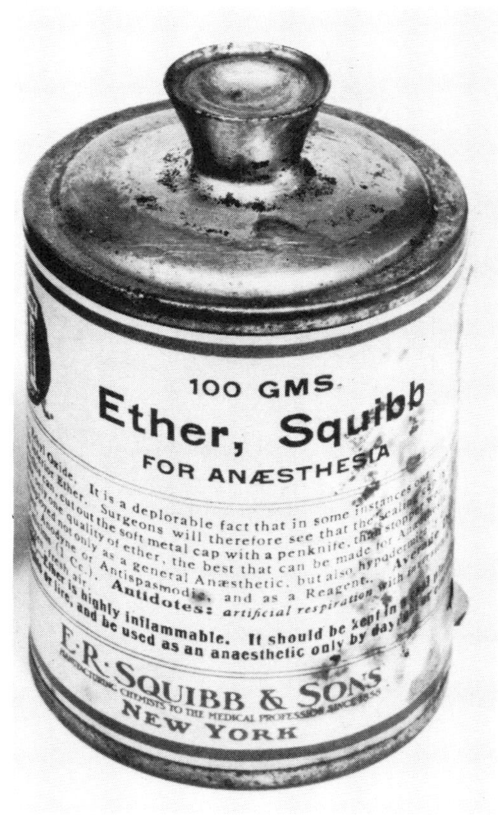

176. OXFORD Vaporizer
c. 1945
An apparatus comprising a cylindrical water bath surrounding an inner container for calcium chloride crystals, which in turn surrounds a chamber for ether. Air is drawn through the apparatus with the patient's inspiration, or may be propelled by compressing the spring-loaded, concertina bellows mounted next to the carrying handle. Gauges for the ether level, temperature of the calcium chloride crystals and the percentage of ether vapour in air (which could be varied) are provided.
The apparatus was devised specifically for military use by R.R. Macintosh (b. 1897) and H.G. Epstein (b. 1909) at Oxford University in 1941 (Epstein *et al.*, 1941). A constant supply of ether vapour was provided by the heat produced on recrystallisation of the calcium chloride crystals. (These were fused initially by several refills of the water bath with hot water – preparations for operation took twenty to thirty minutes (Minnitt and Gillies, 1945: 179)). No gas cylinders were required – an obvious advantage for military use. Engineers from Morris Motors Ltd. were responsible for making the original design suitable for mass production (Nuffield Dept. of Anaesthetics, c. 1942: 12). In 1951 it was still considered the most accurate method available for giving an air-ether mixture, although it had drawbacks for civilian use (Evans, 1951: 92).
310 x 280 mm.
Loaned by The London Hospital, Whitechapel.

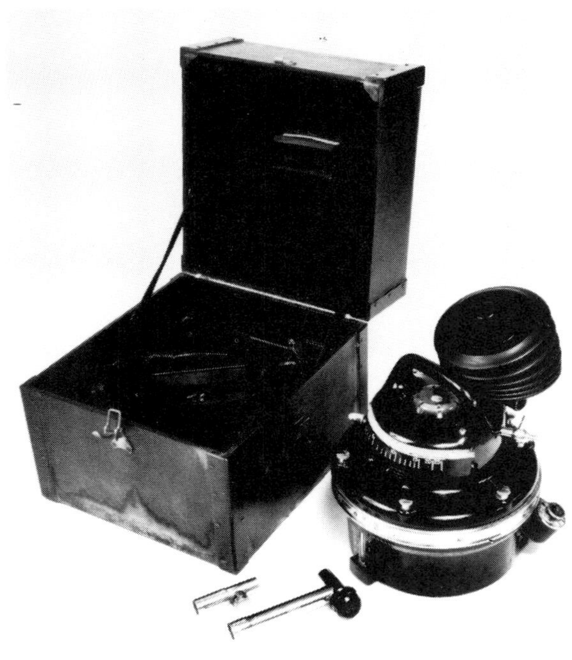

177. OXFORD The Nuffield Department of Anaesthetics, University of Oxford, *The Oxford vaporiser*, [1941?]. A booklet produced by the Oxford department containing instructions for use of the vaporizer and reprints of four articles from *The Lancet* July 19, 1941.

SHOCK

178. FREEZE-DRIED Human Plasma
1982 *SCOTTISH NATIONAL BLOOD TRANS-FUSION SERVICE*
Sealed glass bottle of freeze-dried human plasma, for reconstitution with 400 ml sterile water, with printed label stating that it was prepared from 10 separate donations, and giving expiry date as 20 Sep. 1986.
Under wartime conditions, problems of storing and transporting blood achieved great prominence. Research into the freeze-drying of serum and plasma had begun before the Second World War. The Wellcome Trust provided for a greatly enlarged unit at the Medical Research Council's Cambridge pilot plant in 1942, when it became apparent that the smaller plants of the Wellcome Physiological Research Laboratories, the Army Blood Transfusion Service and the Scottish Transfusion Service were together unable to meet the growing demand. This large scale unit produced 350,000 bottles between 1943 and 1945 (Keynes, 1949: 529).
250 x 74 mm. 1983–395

179. BLOOD transfusion set
c. 1940 *DUFFAUD/PARIS*
A metal case containing a blind-ended glass (now broken) and metal syringe, working capacity 5 ml, with two side connectors, rubber tubing and four needles.

The syringe plunger is grooved. Aligning the groove with the 'donor' connector allows blood to be withdrawn into the syringe. Rotating the barrel through 180 degrees and depressing the plunger expels the blood to the recipient. An inscription on the lid reads, "Regio Esercito Italiano Seringue à transfusion du sang pur du Dr Louis Jube Brevetée S.G.D.G. France et Etranger".
The German and Italian Army Medical Services were both issued with this type of transfusion apparatus during World War Two, "in keeping with the continental predeliction [for direct transfusion]" (Keynes, 1949: 421). This example was found in the Western Desert, c. 1940.
case 159 x 84 x 30 mm. A600460

BARBITURATES

180. EVIPAN SODIUM (Hexobarbitone)
1933–50 *BAYER PRODUCTS LTD/Africa House, Kingsway,/LONDON, W.C.2*
Cardboard carton of five ampoules of sterile distilled water for use with Evipan Sodium, intravenous anaesthetic, each 10.5 ccm. The box originally also contained five ampoules of Evipan Sodium.
Evipan, a short-acting barbiturate, was first used clinically in Germany in 1932 by Helmut Weese (1897–1954). It was subsequently eclipsed by thiopentone, described by John Silas Lundy (1893–1973) of the Mayo Clinic a year later. By 1949, following considerable experience in the Second World War, it was recommended "for humanitarian reasons" as the means of induction, "regardless of the anaesthetic to follow" (Evans, 1951: 198).
box 194 x 98 x 26 mm. A625498

REGIONAL ANALGESIA

181. SPINALS Photographic illustrations demonstrating the use of spinal analgesia in Norman R. James, *Regional analgesia for intra-abdominal surgery*, London, J. & A. Churchill Ltd., 1943, Reprinted 1944, with a foreword by I.W. Magill. James listed ten reasons why spinals with amethocaine hydrochloride should be the anaesthetic of choice in war surgery.

182. ANETHAINE
c. 1950 *Glaxo Laboratories Ltd., Greenford, Middlesex, England*
Corked brown glass bottle containing 1 gram of Anethaine (Amethocaine hydrochloride).
41 x 22 mm. A664831

SPECIAL SERVICES

183. THE NAVY Ronald F. Woolmer, *Anaesthetics afloat*, London, H.K. Lewis, February 1942, reprinted April 1942. Open ether and spinal analgesia were the author's favoured methods.

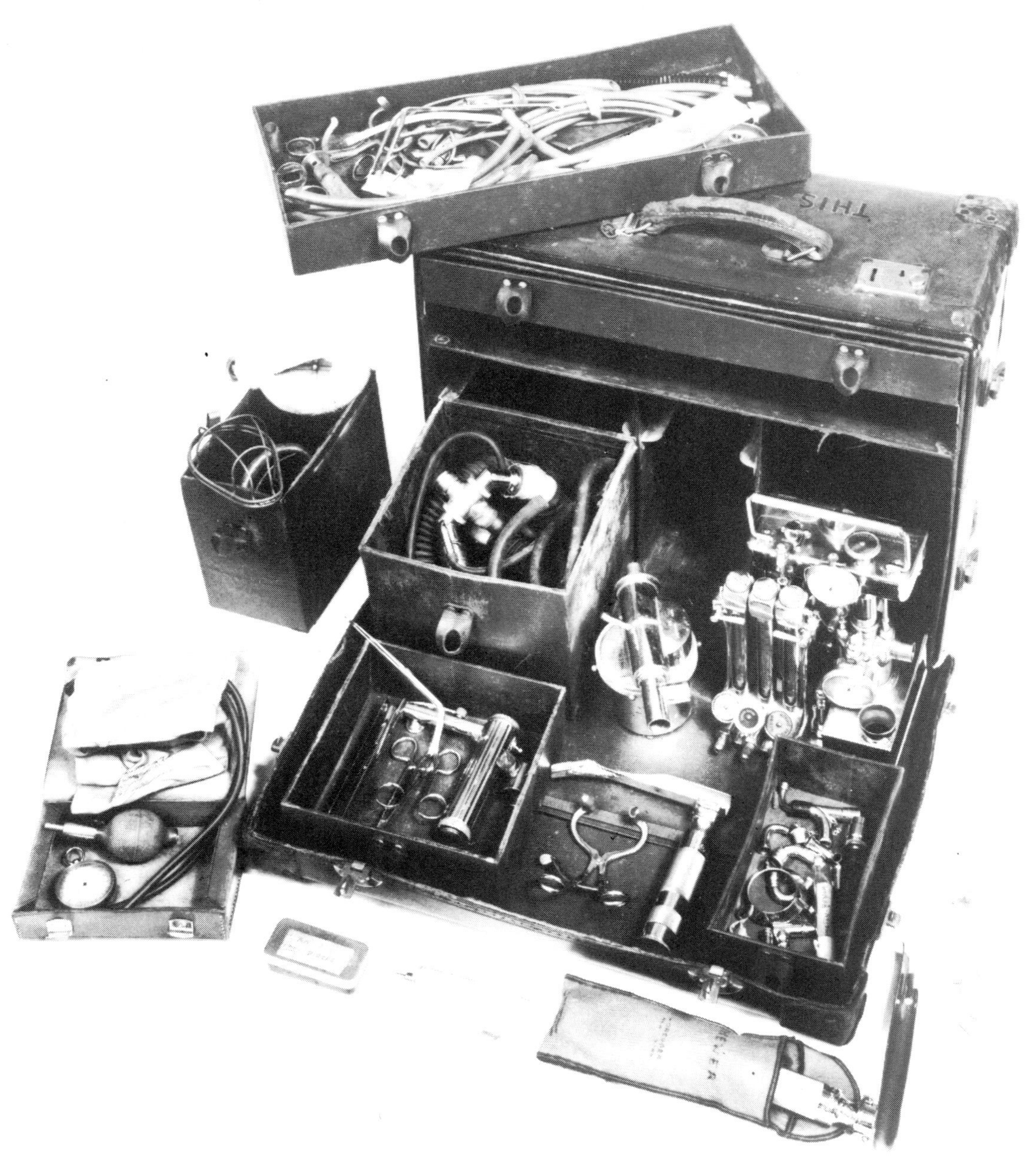

Item 185

As the twentieth century began in Britain, patients undergoing major surgery were generally assured of some form of anaesthetic, very often chloroform (but see Luke 1905: 86–7 for exceptions). No such generalizations, however, can be made about where they would be operated on, or who would anaesthetize them. The confirmation of anaesthesia as a hospital-based specialty, its practitioners awarded equal status with other consultants, came in Britain in 1948 with the creation of the National Health Service. The career of Christopher Langton Hewer (1897–1986), between 1917, when he was first involved, as a medical student, with the anaesthetic department at St. Bartholomew's Hospital, London, and 1961, when he retired from National Health Service practice as a consultant anaesthetist at the same hospital, spans a crucial period of achievement and consolidation for British anaesthetists. Hewer's anaesthetic case, filled with equipment he used between about 1920 and 1950, forms the principal exhibit in this section. This apparatus, with Hewer's own reminiscences (Hewer, 1959), and the recorded details of his career (see e.g. Boulton, 1986; *The Times*, 1986), together provide considerable insight into anaesthesia at a London teaching hospital in the early and middle years of this century.

Hewer qualified in 1918 and considered himself fortunate to be commissioned into a unit of the Royal Army Medical Corps whose anaesthetist was H. Torrance Thomson (1868–1944) of Edinburgh. By 1918, specialist anaesthetists had superseded the general medical officers used in the earlier years of the war (see *Anaesthesia and Two World Wars*). Hewer returned to St. Bartholomew's in 1919 as Assistant Administrator of Anaesthetics, becoming Administrator of Anaesthetics at the age of 28 (*The Times*, 1986). The hospital was unusual in having maintained an unbroken line of specialist anaesthetic appointments since 1852 (Scurr, 1971: 279). Elsewhere in Britain, especially outside London, anaesthetics were still given by medical practitioners with no special experience, or by unqualified assistants (see e.g. Page, 1984: 114–5). Repeated attempts were made from 1908 onwards to bring about legislation restricting the administration of anaesthetics to medical practitioners (Scurr, 1971: 276–8). Proposed legislation perished in the turmoil of 1914, but after the war pressure for better anaesthetic training facilities increased in strength. Like his contemporaries, Hewer himself had received no formal, postgraduate education in anaesthetics, since none was available. There were, however, two established British textbooks – D.J. Buxton's *Anaesthetics* (1888) and F.J. Hewitt's *Anaesthetics and their administration* (1893). Both went through numerous editions, in each case the last, in 1920 and 1922, respectively, was almost twice the size of the first. It seems likely that Hewitt was not superseded in popularity in Britain until after J.A. Lee's *Synopsis of anaesthesia* was published in 1946. Hewer specifically acknowledged his debt to Hewitt's book (Hewer 1959: 312).

An adjunct to textbooks, in the shape of formal tuition for doctors in anaesthesiology, was begun in the United States, in 1928, when R. M. Waters (1883–1979) instituted postgraduate fellowships at the University of Wisconsin (Scurr, 1979: 289; Rupreht, 1985: 33). Formal assessment of training in anaesthesia came first in Britain, with the creation of a Diploma in Anaesthetics in 1935. The Association of Anaesthetists of Great Britain and Ireland was founded, in 1932, partly to achieve this end. The only organized professional body for anaesthetists in Britain prior to this was the Section of Anaesthetics of the Royal Society of Medicine (Scurr, 1979: 282). Hewer became a founder member of the new Association. In the same year, he edited the first volume of *Recent advances in anaesthesia and analgesia* (Hewer, 1932) and remained editor of the series for the next half century. The appearance of the *Recent advances* series, specifically *not* designed as an elementary textbook, was indicative of a growing perception that anaesthesia was indeed a theory-based medical specialty. In certain circles, however, it was still regarded as a practical and empirical discipline. British anaesthesia acquired its first professorial chair, at the University of Oxford, somewhat earlier than might otherwise have occurred through the direct intervention of the industrialist, William Morris, later Lord Nuffield (1877–1963). Only by making the endowment, in 1937, of chairs in medicine, surgery and obstetrics conditional on the creation of one in anaesthesia did Nuffield succeed in changing the University's opinion that the creation of a chair in such a subject as anaesthetics would expose them to ridicule (Rupreht, 1985: 355).

A certain resistance to the provision of postgraduate anaesthetic training was encountered among anaesthetists themselves in this period. As R.R. Macintosh (b. 1897) (first incumbent of the Oxford chair) later remarked, "few of the seniors went out of their way to encourage promising juniors who might well become rivals in the highly competitive private practice which was after all their only source of livelihood" (quoted in Scurr, 1979: 284). This was a factor which directly influenced several aspects of anaesthetic practice. Hewer's hospital appointment, like those of his colleagues, was honorary until 1948, and one feature of his apparatus – portability – was related to the necessity of anaesthetizing private patients in their own houses, or in one of the increasing number of private surgical nursing homes opened during the 1920s and 30s. Anaesthetic carrying cases with suggested lists, not of equipment for emergencies, but for comprehensive surgical anaesthesia, featured in manufacturers' catalogues during the 1930s and 40s (see e.g. Down Bros., Ltd., 1935: 1325–6A). Often these cases incorporated compartments for gas cylinders.

At St. Bartholomew's, the need for the anaesthetist, or hospital, to supply cylinders (other than in emergencies) began to be obviated during 1930, when a system of piped gases was installed in the new surgical block (Hewer, 1959: 320). This was only one of many changes in equipment and technique which Hewer witnessed during his career at Bart's. Recalling anaesthetic practice there as he had first known it in 1917, Hewer describes a scene dominated by Victorian equipment – including Hewitt's gas and air apparatus, and Clover's inhaler for major surgery in adults – into which the introduction of a replica of the Gwathmey machine, constructed at the request of H.E.G. Boyle (1895–1941), caused considerable excitement (Hewer, 1959: 312–4). The demands of new surgical techniques, at their most complex in the teaching hospitals, were a motor for change in anaesthetic practice in the years between the wars. Hewer, through the special interests of various surgeons at Bart's, was particularly involved with thyroid and with thoracic surgery. As an anaesthetist however, he still had only limited autonomy. He recalled that in the 1920s endotracheal tubes were used under facemasks, hidden from surgeons who considered that they caused tracheitis.

As the war ended, British anaesthetists were anticipating and actively preparing for the reorganization of health care that was to come in 1948. The 1947 issue of the journal of the Association of Anaesthetists, *Anaesthesia*, which Hewer edited for twenty years from its foundation in 1946, used the occasion of the centenary of anaesthesia to impress upon public and profession alike, the "increasing sophistication of the work of the anaesthetist" (Boulton, 1977: 898). Links with the surgeons were formalized in 1948, a Faculty of Anaesthetists being created in the Royal College of Surgeons of England. Equal status and remuneration with other hospital consultants was duly achieved at the creation of the National Health Service. Before the war, in 1938, there were 86 consultant anaesthetists in Great Britain. By 1962, the year after Hewer's retirement from the NHS, the figure was over ten times higher (Boulton, 1964: 304).

GENERAL SURGERY

184. PHOTOGRAPH of the surgeon, George Grey Turner (1877–1951) operating in Newcastle, March 1940. The anaesthetist is using a gas and oxygen machine.

185. C. LANGTON HEWER'S ANAESTHETIC CASE
1920–60 Various makers, especially A. Charles King. A leather carrying case with six drawers of anaesthetic equipment, a compartment housing Hewer's own design of continuous flow gas and oxygen apparatus, with a carbon dioxide absorber, and a sphygmomanometer and Foregger laryngoscope in individual cases. Two stoppered glass bottles, with typescript labels '$C_2HClBrF_3$', the chemical formula for halothane, are included.
Hewer's continuous flow gas and oxygen apparatus was made by A. Charles King and resembled Lewis's machine, which Hewer was recommending in 1932 for endotracheal anaesthesia (Hewer, 1932: 77–8). It incorporates an ether dropper with variable rate, above a vaporizing chamber in a water-bath heated by a spirit lamp. This apparatus found favour with other authors during the 1940s (see e.g. Minnitt and Gillies, 1945: 185).

Amongst the smaller items are cuffed endotracheal tubes – for some years Hewer was under the misapprehension that he had invented the pilot bulb, to indicate deflation of the cuff (Hewer, 1959: 318) – and a Clausen's rubber head harness, used in Hewer's method of anaesthetizing patients with toxic goitre, to hold a facemask in place (Hewer, 1932: 143–4).
590 x 250 x 490 mm.
Loaned by Dr. David Wilkinson, St. Bartholomew's Hospital.

186. TRILENE
c. 1945 *IMPERIAL CHEMICAL (PHARMACEUTICALS) LTD/MANCHESTER*
Two boxes containing five 6 cc ampoules of 'Trilene' for inhalation.
Trichlorethylene, first described in 1864, was studied by German neurologists in the 1920s and 1930s. This stimulated research in the USA into its potential as a useful anaesthetic agent (Ostlere, 1953: 1–13). In Britain in 1939 it was recommended, by a chemist, to the Joint Committee of the Medical Research Council and the Section of Anaesthetics of the Royal Society of Medicine, of which Hewer was a member. This group was seeking a non-flammable anaesthetic for wartime use. Hewer began cautious trials at St. Bartholomew's Hospital, London, in 1940, having found that trichlorethylene was already marketed

as a cleansing agent for wounds and had been used as a solvent in heavy industry (Hewer, 1942: 463–4). It was made by ICI under the trade name 'Trilene' and the company, at Hewer's suggestion, added 'waxolene blue' dye to distinguish the new agent from chloroform. Hewer became a firm supporter of the drug (Hewer, 1959: 321–3).
box 122 x 90 x 27 mm. 1986–1660

187. HALOTHANE
1980 MAY & BAKER LTD DAGENHAM
Supplied in a 250 ml brown glass screw topped bottle, with printed paper label.
Halothane was introduced in 1956 in Britain, a result of the postwar search for a safe, potent, nonexplosive volatile anaesthetic. Its success in Britain has been attributed to its easy adaptation to the Boyle's machine, and to the organization of the British health services after 1948, whereby anaesthetists did not have to meet the cost of anaesthetic agents used, except in private practice (Halothane was relatively expensive) (Stephen and Little, 1961:105). Hewer, nearing retirement, initially was not keen on the new agent (Hewer, 1959:328).
150 x 70 mm. 1981–706

RESUSCITATION

188. FREDERIC W. HEWITT *Anaesthetics and their administration*, 2nd ed., London, Macmillan and Co. Ltd., 1901, fig. 12, p. 200, 'Emergency Case, containing Mason's gag, Tongue-forceps, Wooden Wedge, Mouth-prop, Instruments for performing Tracheotomy, Hypodermic Syringe, and partition for remedies such as Nitrite of Amyl, Digitalis, Strychnine, etc.'. Tracheotomy was preferred to intubation in respiratory emergencies well into the twentieth century.

189. CHAMPAGNE Brut
n.d. (Non-vintage) *Veuve Clicquot Ponsardin.*
If vomiting was a complication after ether administration Dudley Buxton recommended that "iced dry champagne may be given in teaspoonful doses every quarter of an hour until improvement occurs" (Buxton, 1907: 176). It was no longer recommended by the fifth edition of 1914.
750 ml.

190. MORPHINE
1862–3 W.N. Walton
Shop round with glass-fronted phototype label: Sol. Morph. Mur. (Crellin and Scott 1972: 45). "The hypodermic injection of $\frac{1}{6}$ grain of morphine may also be of great use in cases of persistent [laryngeal] spasm" (Gardner, 1916: 26).
210 x 75 mm. A633823

191. NUX VOMICA
1902–28 SAVORY & MOORE LTD,/29 Chapel Street,/LONDON S.W.1. In hexagonal glass bottle with ribbed back and printed paper label.

Nux vomica, or its active constituent, strychnine, remained a recommended treatment for post-anaesthetic shock until well into the twentieth century (e.g. Nosworthy, 1935: 40).
150 x 49 mm. A642367

192. 'VAPOROLE' of Amyl Nitrite
c. 1931 *BURROUGHS WELLCOME & CO/ (THE WELLCOME FOUNDATION LTD.)/ LONDON (ENG.)*
Box containing twelve amyl nitrite capsules. Vaporole was a Burroughs Wellcome & Co. Trade Mark. Buxton recommended amyl nitrite in cases of 'syncope' after chloroform administration (Buxton, 1907: 245) (see *Anaesthesia and the Chloroform Question*). Hewitt considered it, together with strychnine, the "most reliable" drug for dealing with "alarming symptoms" (Hewitt, 1901: 201).
57 x 40 x 15 mm. WFA LEN/45

193. 'VAPOROLE' of Aromatic Ammonia
c. 1914 *BURROUGHS WELLCOME & CO./ LONDON (ENG)*
Box containing 12 capsules of aromatic ammonia in silk "sacs". 'Smelling salts' were recommended after chloroform overdosage (Silk, 1920: 131).
57 x 40 x 15 mm. WFA EN/45

194. ASPHYXIA H. Bellamy Gardner, *The asphyxial factor in anaesthesia and other essays*, London, Baillière, Tindall and Cox, 1901. A treatise on the management of special anaesthetic problems.

THE PROFESSION

195. TEXTBOOKS Five editions of Dudley W. Buxton's textbook *Anaesthetics. Their uses and administration.* From the first (1888) to the fifth (1914) (see Bibliography). A sixth edition appeared in 1920 and was reprinted several times. In 1888 Buxton was "Administrator of anaesthetics at University College Hospital" (t.p.).

196. REFORM Frederic W. Hewitt, *The position of the present reform movement in anaesthetics*, London, John Bale, Sons & Danielsson, 1911. Reprinted from *The Lancet*, 1911, *i*: 1486–9, 1562–5. Inscribed "Prof. W.D. Halliburton F.R.S. with the author's compliments".

197. REFORM Photographs of Bills proposed to regulate the administration of anaesthetics, in 1909 (Bills 120 and 259). (House of Commons Library)

198. C. LANGTON HEWER, *Recent advances in anaesthesia and analgesia*, London, J. & A. Churchill, 1932. The first volume of a series which Hewer edited for fifty years.

199. JOURNALS *Anaesthesia,* 1946, *1* (1). The first issue of the Journal of the Association of Anaesthetists. The *British Journal of Anaesthesia*, had first appeared in 1923, and the American journal *Current researches in anesthesia and analgesia* in 1920.

CASE 11: ANAESTHESIA AND INDUSTRY: ONE

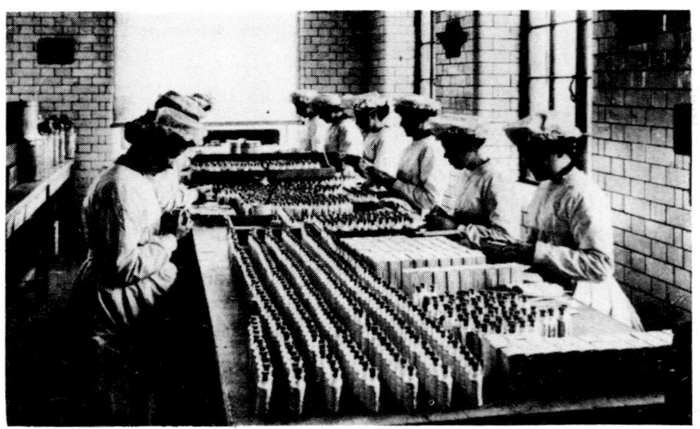

Item 209

The increasing dependence of the practice of anaesthesia on industry has received only erratic attention from historians. By far the greatest scrutiny has been given to the early problems of medical gas production (Smith, 1982). Studies on the development and production of non-gaseous anaesthetic agents in the context of the fine chemical and pharmaceutical industry as a whole, and on the research, development and marketing of anaesthetic apparatus by the medical equipment industry, have not been pursued to any extent.

Increasing demand for nitrous oxide in the 1870s, and the problems associated with the distribution and purity of the gas, made centralized, large scale production potentially profitable at a time when ether and chloroform continued to be produced on the premises of pharmacists. Originally supplied in cumbersome bladders or bags, nitrous oxide was, by 1868, available compressed into iron bottles from the British firms of George Barth and Coxeter & Son. From 1870, liquid gas was supplied (Smith, 1982: 133–4). Distribution costs became much higher than production costs for medical gases. Most companies preferred to retain ownership of cylinders and valves, doing business on the basis of exchanging full cylinders for empty. The piping of gases from a central source, often in the basement of hospitals, began early this century in America. Other countries slowly followed suit, although the movement of heavy, bulky cylinders in emergency remained a feature of hospital life and company policy – most offered next day delivery as routine, with a faster service available at extra cost. Recent figures for the supply of oxygen to the non-medical and medical markets indicate that distribution costs remain a major factor. A British steelworks in 1971 consumed in a fortnight the amount of oxygen used in British medicine in a year, at similar levels of purity. But, for the widely scattered medical market the distribution cost of gas in cylinders, per cubic foot, was as much as two hundred times that for gas piped directly to steelworks (Ouvry, 1971).

By the time large scale manufacture of non-gaseous anaesthetic drugs began, the British chemical industry was in relative decline. The early achievements of the industrial revolution had been based on the production of inorganics. Initial priority in organic chemicals, particularly dye stuffs, was quickly lost to Germany. By 1913, Britain ranked a poor third to this country and the United States in terms of the world chemical market (Roderick and Stephens, 1981: 156). Historians differ in the reasons they proffer for Britain's decline. Idiosyncrasies of the patenting system, failure to invest in research and a lack of trained engineers to run plant have all been cited (Ibid.: 163). Whatever its cause, the decline ensured that in anaesthetics, as in other drugs, innovation was predominantly German in the late nineteenth and early twentieth century. Cocaine (1884), the less toxic procaine (1905) and the barbiturates (from 1903) are examples here. Between the wars, initiative moved to the United States. In the 1930s the introduction of the new gaseous agent, cyclopropane, involved close co-operation between the Ohio Chemical Company, basic scientists and anaesthetists. The high cost of this agent was to affect directly the design of anaesthetic equipment. 'Closed-circuit' techniques, in which the patient rebreathed expired air and anaesthetic gases (with carbon dioxide removed) cut down the amount of anaesthetic agent used and also the explosion risk (cyclopropane was highly flammable) (Rupreht, 1982: 271–5). Systematic laboratory research, funded by major pharmaceutical firms, has been the source of new anaesthetic drugs since the 1950s. Chemists have used theories of molecular structure to predict potentially useful agents. Synthesis of hundreds of fluorocarbons in ICI's Pharmaceutical Laboratories resulted in the introduction of the highly successful 'fluothane' in 1956 (Rupreht, 1982: 289).

Anaesthetic equipment featured in surgical instrument manufacturers' catalogues from the 1850s. Until well into the twentieth century, despite the industrialization of production techniques, and the gradual demise of the inventive, specialist instrument maker (of whom perhaps A. Charles King (1888–1966) was the foremost example in anaesthetics), considerable liason continued to occur between individual anaesthetists and manufacturers, as in the case of Coxeter's co-operation with H.E.G. Boyle (1895–1941) in producing his now famous machine (Watt, 1968: 104). Innovation continued to come from individual anaesthetists, who remained the main customers. A radical change in the market for anaesthetic equipment came about in Britain with the creation of the National Health Service in 1948, although the trend toward hospital provision of anaesthetic equipment, increasingly expensive and complex and decreasingly portable, had already begun. Boyle's machine was originally designed as a portable apparatus and was advertised packed in carrying cases throughout the 1930s and 40s, alongside hospital models. After 1950 the portable models are rarely found.

Measures to standardize anaesthetic equipment, at which there had been various international attempts following World War Two, now became the subject of government regulation in National Health Service hospitals. In 1955, the mandatory introduction of non-interchangeable couplings between gas cylinder and flowmeter (see *Monitoring in Anaesthesia*) to prevent the wrong gas being given to the patient, was an example of such legislation, which required extensive co-operation between manufacturers and hospitals (Watt, 1968: 113). In recent years, the whole of the medical equipment industry has had to turn its attention to satisfying the regulations of other countries – a lengthy and expensive procedure, but an essential one in securing international markets on which profitability now depends.

SURGICAL GASES

200. GAS HOLDER
1850–1900
A painted zinc receiver with brass carrying handles and high domed base. A metal tube conveys gas to the space between the receiver wall and the top of the dome, where it is trapped beneath an outer cover. The latter rises above a water seal, assisted by a weighted pulley mechanism (missing from this example, the finish of which has been restored).
Prior to 1868, nitrous oxide had to be made as required, or purchased in bladders or bags. Gas holders were used to collect the gas as it was made (often by heating ammonium nitrate). After 1868, compressed (and later liquified) nitrous oxide became available in cylinders (Smith, 1982: 123–53). These were often connected to fill a portable gasometer (see e.g. Buxton, 1892: 46). According to Luke, the gasometer was seldom used by 1905, "being expensive, apt to leak and get out of order" and "the reverse of the portable" (Luke, 1905: 17).
445 x 340 mm. A631300

201. NITROUS OXIDE Illustration of 'Gasometer and inhaler' for preparing and administering nitrous oxide in Laurence Turnbull, *Artificial anaesthesia*, Philadelphia, P. Blakiston, Son & Co., 1896, p. 42.

202. NITROUS OXIDE CYLINDER
c. 1870
Bulbous copper cylinder with brazed bands and brass tap. The firm of Barth were said to have supplied similar quart-size cylinders containing fifteen gallons of gas "so the pressure in them was really below the limits of safety and in more than one instance the end blew off" (Shuter, 1912, quoted in Smith, 1982: 134).
340 x 137 mm. A625424

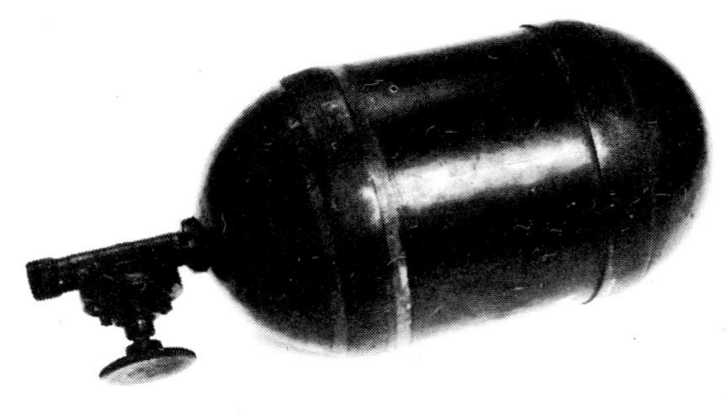

203. NITROUS OXIDE CYLINDERS
1935 *G. BARTH & Co*
Two cylinders for liquid nitrous oxide, with side valves and brass union. Hewitt favoured working with two cylinders "in case one should work badly or fall short during the administration". The average amount required was six gallons per patient (Hewitt, 1901: 209, 213). Barth & Co. had developed a valve which did not freeze up when the cylinders were used horizontally, with a foot key (Ibid.: 210).
290 x 156 mm. A625426

204. NITROUS OXIDE CYLINDER
1939 *THE/BRITISH OXYGEN CO. LTD./
WEMBLEY/MIDDLESEX*
Iron, round-bottomed 25 gall. cylinder with brass
tap and printed paper label stating that it was filled
2 January, 1939. The British Standard Specification
('BSS NO 401/1931') is moulded on the cylinder base.
The British Oxygen Co. Ltd., founded 1906, relied on
the market for oxygen created by limelight, and then
by oxyacetylene blowpipes – it did not have a medical
division until 1937 (Smith, 1982: xxv). In 1925, the
company was manufacturing nitrous oxide in Wemb-
ley and Manchester for anaesthetic use, and offered a
'Free London Motor Delivery Service' (Smith, 1982:
145). When a medical division opened, they undertook to make every effort to "execute urgent orders
received by telegram from medical men" out of working hours (BOC, c. 1937: 9).
286 x 114 mm. A662293

205. PHOTOGRAPH of a surgical operation at the
Middlesex Hospital, c. 1928.

CHLOROFORM AND ETHER

206. 'VAPOROLES' of chloroform
c. 1897 *Burroughs, Wellcome & Co.*
Cardboard box containing 10 chloroform capsules
(and space for two more), with accompanying leaflet.
The Company marketed chloroform and ether for respiratory difficulties. They were supplied in capsules,
enclosed in cotton wool in a silk bag. These were to
be crushed, dropped in a jug of hot water and the
vapour inhaled.
90 x 75 x 44 mm. WFA EN/45

207. 'VAPOROLES' of ether
c. 1897 *Burroughs, Wellcome & Co.*
Cardboard box containing 12 capsules of ether.
90 x 75 x 44 mm. WFA EN/45

208. WELLCOME
(a) Copy of a letter from Duncan, Flockhart
& Co., Edinburgh, to Burroughs Wellcome & Co.,
London, informing them of the price of chloroform,
January 17, 1903. (WFA D3 Chloroform)
(b) Memorandum from Burroughs Wellcome
& Co., London, to J.F. Macfarlane & Co., London,
asking for "your closest quotation for pure chloroform" and "the minimum quantity that must be taken
in order to secure rock bottom prices", January 15,
1903. At this time Wellcome were using the chloroform to make 'vaporoles'. Only in 1906 did they begin
to advertise that they were manufacturing and selling
it as an anaesthetic. (WFA D3 Chloroform)

209. PHOTOGRAPH of the Wellcome Chemical
Works, Dartford, c. 1909.

210. PHOTOGRAPH of an advertisement for 'Wellcome Brand Chloroform', *The Chemist and Druggist*,
1916, Feb. 12: 31. It was supplied in bottles and "her-
metically sealed" tubes. Wellcome chloroform cost 3s
10d per pound, in a bottle.

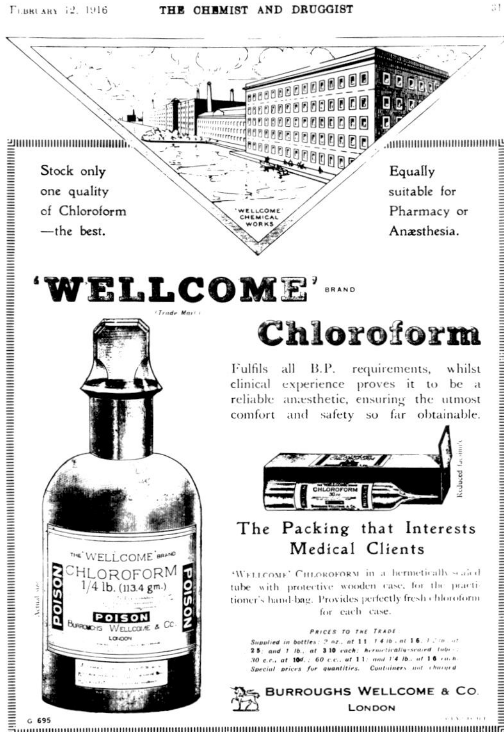

211. DUNCAN *The history of Duncan, Flockhart
& Co. commemorating the centenaries of ether and
chloroform*, Edinburgh, Duncan, Flockhart & Co.,
1946. The business was founded in Perth, Scotland,
in 1806, by a druggist John Duncan (1780–1871).
Duncan supplied Simpson with his first batch of chloroform in 1847, and much of the company's subsequent success was built on the manufacture of the
drug. (WMSM)

212. DUNCAN Duncan, Flockhart & Co., *General
index and price current*, Edinburgh, Duncan, Flockhart & Co., 1938–9, p. 39. Advertisement for the company's three varieties of chloroform.

ETHYL CHLORIDE

213. ETHYL CHOLRIDE
1925–40 *DUNCAN, FLOCKHART & COMP./
Edinburgh and London.*
Absolute Ethyl Chloride, sp. gr. 0.920, supplied in a
60cc glass cylinder, with printed paper scale. The
metal nozzle was designed to produce a coarse spray
which could be applied to a fabric facemask.
Ethyl chloride is a vapour at normal pressure and
temperature and was filled into special tubes under
pressure. It was "accepted" in clinical practice after 1896 (Duncum, 1947: 498–516). In the twentieth
century it came to be considered more suitable for
inducing, rather than maintaining, anaesthesia. The
agent was also used to produce local anaesthesia (by
refrigeration).
case 192 x 34 mm. A625482

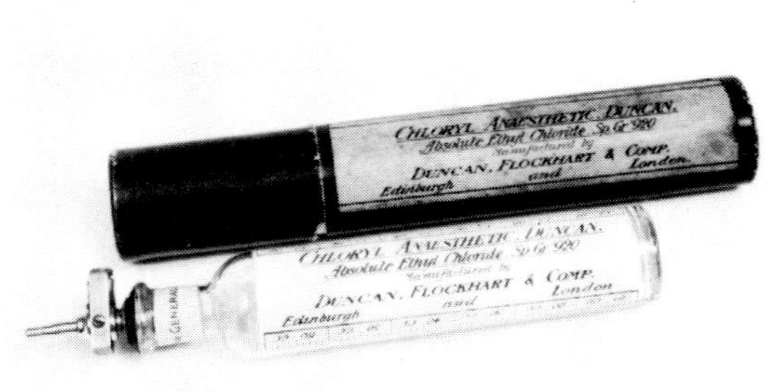

214. CATALOGUE Duncan, Flockhart & Co., *Medical Catalogue*, Edinburgh, Duncan, Flockhart & Co., 1946, p. 33 'Ethyl Chloride'. The catalogue advertised 30cc, 60cc and 100cc tubes. The 60cc tube cost 5 shillings. Perfumed ethyl chloride for use with children could also be purchased. (WMSM)

BARBITURATES

215. PENTOTHAL Abbott Laboratories Ltd., *Pentothal*, c. 1953. Promotional booklet. Pentothal was the registered trademark for the barbiturate Thiopentone Sodium B.P. Pentothal was marketed as an induction agent, as an adjunct to any other drug, and as a primary anaesthetic. It was introduced in 1934 (Rupreht, 1985: 88–91).

216. PHOTOGRAPH of an advertisement for Brevital in *Anesthesiology*, 1962, *23*: 47. Brevital, made by Lilly, was an "ultrashort-acting intravenous barbiturate", marketed for its "Quick smooth induction" and "Safe, more clearheaded recovery".

MUSCLE RELAXANTS

217. INTOCOSTRIN E.R. Squibb & Sons, *Intocostrin*, c. 1945. Promotional booklet. Intocostrin, a curare preparation, was marketed as an intravenous muscle relaxant and promoted primarily for "softening the severity of the convulsions and preventing fractures" in "the shock therapy of mental disease" (p. 3). "Curarization" with intocostrin was regarded as sufficient preparation. No anaesthetic agent, either intravenous or inhalational, was advised. It was recommended that an "airflow" be kept available (p. 9). (Loaned by Dr. David Wilkinson)

218. TUBARINE *d-Tubocurarine chloride. Supplementary notes on the documentary film produced by the Wellcome Film Unit*, [1948]. Wellcome marketed Tubarine, an intramuscular curare preparation, for muscle relaxation during surgery and shock therapy. In the latter instance thiopentone was recommended as the anaesthetic of choice. (Loaned by Dr. David Wilkinson)

219. TUBARINE
1946 *Burroughs Wellcome & Co., LONDON*.
Carton of six ampoules containing Tubarine, (d-Tubocurarine chloride), a crystalline extract of tube

curare, found by some workers in 1944 to be of more reliable potency than intocostrin (Gray and Halton, 1946: 401). By 1949, one anaesthetist considered it likely that the muscle relaxants had 'inaugurated yet another stage of progress towards perfection in the art and science of anaesthesia" (Evans, 1951: 18). 84 x 63 x 18 mm. A642913

220. ELECTRO-CONVULSIVE Therapy machine 1945 *SPENCER PATERSON*
A headband to hold two padded electrodes connected to a multiple tap transformer via a voltage selector switch and a telephone dial acting as a mechanical timer. Another secondary winding provides a voltage for resistance readings across the head. The whole apparatus, Mark IV, serial no. 244, is fitted in a wooden carrying case (for a survey of the design of this type of apparatus prior to 1949, see MacPhail, 1949: 33–6). Some of the earliest clinical trials of intravenous intocostrin (an extract of d-tubocurarine of known potency) involved its use in the prevention of trauma in a series of patients undergoing electro-convulsive therapy (Gray and Halton, 1946: 400). 320 x 147 x 236 mm. 1984–159

OXYGEN

221. THERAPY British Oxygen Gases Ltd., *Oxygen Therapy*, 1959. Booklet produced to advertise oxygen therapy equipment. The large scale marketing of oxygen as a therapy, as well as an adjunct to anaesthetic gases, occurred after the Second World War. (Loaned by Dr. David Wilkinson)

222. PHOTOGRAPH produced for promotional purposes, by the British Oxygen Company, showing delivery of its gas cylinders to a dental surgery c. 1955. (Loaned by Dr. David Wilkinson)

223. STANDARDS The British Oxygen Co. Ltd., *Oxygen therapy equipment*, c. 1955, p. 36. Showing 'British standard colours for medical gas cylinders'. Large scale supply of equipment and standard parts were a post-World War Two phenomenon. In Britain, standard colours for gas cylinders were introduced in 1955. (WMSM)

OPIUM

224. OMNOPON Roche Products Ltd., *Omnopon*, c. 1939? Omnopon, known as Pantopon in America, was and is a proprietary name for a water soluble extract containing all the opium alkaloids. It was introduced early in this century and was marketed for pain relief, pre-medication and, with scopolamine, for use in 'twilight sleep' (see *Anaesthesia and Women*). (Loaned by Dr. David Wilkinson)

225. PHOTOGRAPH showing 'sealing Omnopon Ampoules' at the Roche Plant, Welwyn Garden City, England. (From the booklet described above)

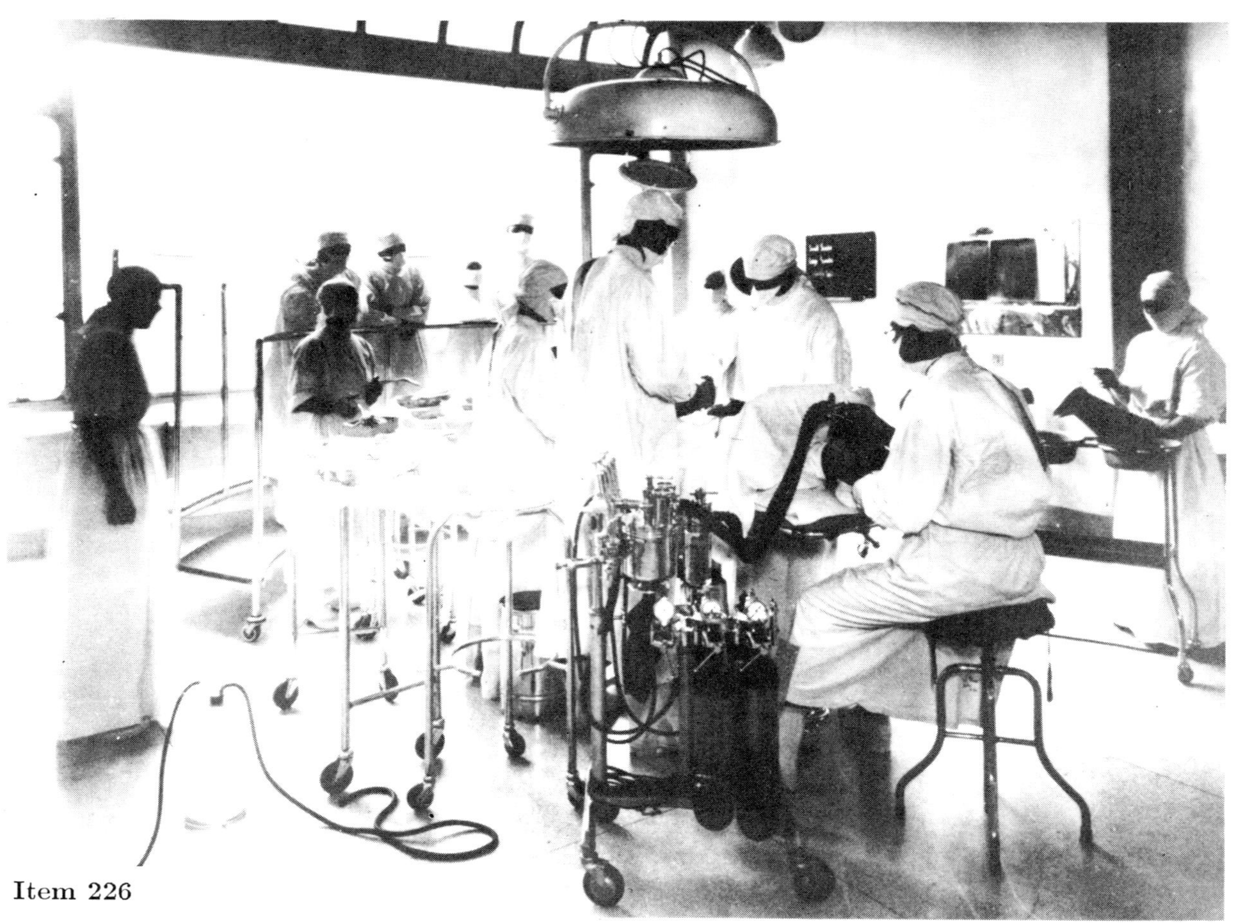

Item 226

GAS AND OXYGEN

226. PHOTOGRAPH of an operation at Park Hospital, London, c. 1955. (Copyright of the Greater London Photographic Library 80/7392)

227. GAS-OXYGEN Apparatus
1931–8 *ALLEN & HANBURYS/LTD./LONDON.*
Apparatus comprising two 100 gallon nitrous oxide cylinders and one 30 gallon oxygen cylinder, with a central metal stand to support facepiece, tubing, and a clear glass gas mixing bottle. Both gases were bubbled through water in this bottle by means of separate, perforated tubes "enabling the proportions to be adjusted as required" (Allen and Hanbury's, 1938: 23). A respiration indicator, rebreathing bag, and three facemasks together with one for nasal administration, are included. In 1938, the total cost of the outfit, packed in a brown fibre box with carrying handle and weighing 50lbs, was ten guineas.
Not all anaesthetists took up the use of 'gas and oxygen' for major surgery with equal enthusiasm. Blomfield considered the method to have "received an unnatural impulse during the Great War", the "great success ... in war surgery" having "swung the pendulum of favour rather too widely in civil practice" (Blomfield, 1922: 177–8). Inconveniences continued to be noted in the 1940s, including outlay and running costs and unsuitability for a "beginner" (Minnitt and Gillies, 1945: 115).
672 x 361 x 200 mm. A630961

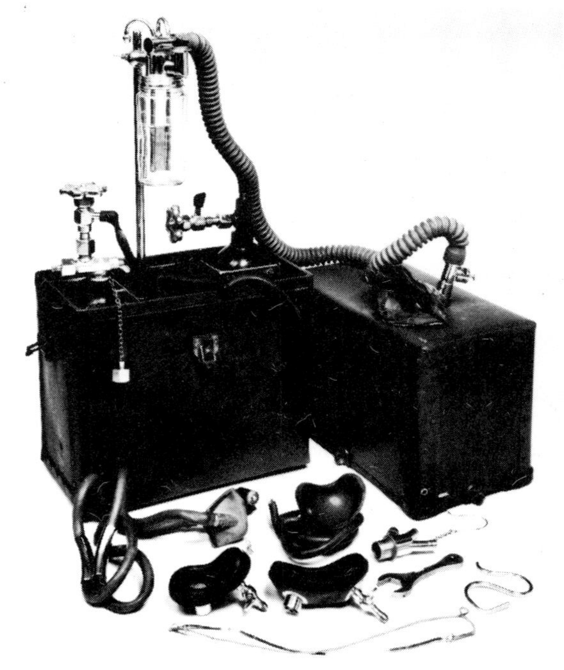

228. BOYLE'S APPARATUS Medical & Industrial Equipment, Ltd., *General anaesthesia apparatus. Hospital Boyle type models*, c. 1960. Trade Catalogue.

229. BOYLE'S APPARATUS British Oxygen Company Limited, *Boyle anaesthetic apparatus*, 1967. Trade Catalogue. The catalogue describes a 'pipeline' model, for use with piped hospital gases, a feature increasingly employed in the 1960s (compare the mobility of anaesthetic apparatus in *Anaesthesia and a New Century*).

230. BOYLE'S APPARATUS British Oxygen Company, Medical, *Boyle International*, January 1974. Trade Catalogue.

NEW AGENTS

231. CYCLOPROPANE
1940–55 *E.R. SQUIBB & SONS, NEW YORK*
Two 'amplon' bottles of liquified cyclopropane gas, with piercing block and key for opening. The cylinders are of a light metal alloy, liquefaction of cyclopropane gas occurring at relatively low pressures. The anaesthetic use of cyclopropane, first synthesized in 1882, was the result of collaboration between anaesthetists and basic scientists, principally at Wisconsin General Hospital, Madison, U.S.A. from 1930. Its relative expense ($2.50 per US gall), owing to small scale production hampered research during the Depression (Rupreht, 1985: 271–5). In the USA it was later to be produced cheaply from propane, a by-product of the oil industry (Evans, 1951: 73). In Britain it remained expensive – 2s–9d a gallon in 1945 (Minnitt and Gillies, 1945: 142). The use of "closed circuit" techniques reduced anaesthetic costs (see the essay in *Anaesthesia and Industry: One*). By 1951, it was considered not to have "fulfilled its early promise" (Evans, 1951: 126), but was of special value in complex procedures, such as chest surgery.
bottles 70 x 30 mm. 1987–406

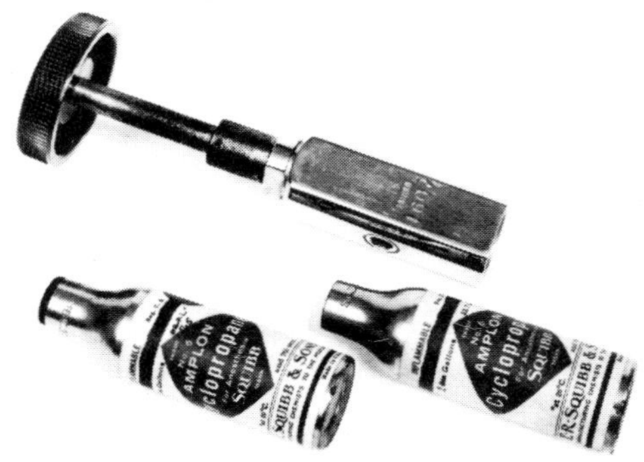

232. VINESTHENE Pharmaceutical Specialities (May & Baker) Ltd., *Vinesthene*, n.d., c. 1938. An advertising booklet describing Vinesthene, the May & Baker preparation of vinyl ether. It was first used clinically in 1933 and was marketed as an agent for short anaesthesias. It could be given by the drop method, by an inhaler or incorporated into a gas and oxygen circuit. In c. 1938 a 25cc bottle cost 4s–6d. (Loaned by Dr. David Wilkinson)

233. VINESTHENE (Divinyl Ether)
1951–2 *MAY & BAKER LTD./DAGENHAM ENG-LAND*
Supplied in a 25cc brown glass bottle, with printed label giving instructions to place on ice before opening when using at temperatures above 70deg.F.
A volatile liquid anaesthetic. Its high volatility, instability and cost largely restricted its use to rapid (1–3 minute) anaesthetics given by means of a single dose (Wylie and Churchill-Davidson, 1972: 311).
90 x 30 mm.
Loaned by Dr. David Wilkinson, St. Bartholomew's Hospital.

234. V.A.M. (Divynyl Ether Mixture)
1940–60 *MAY & BAKER LTD. DAGENHAM ENG-LAND*
A 4oz glass bottle of 'V.A.M. anaesthetic mixture' in grey paper packaging with printed label.
V.A.M. was a mixture of 25% Vinesthene and 75% ethyl ether. An attempt to produce a less volatile and irritating vapour than that of pure ether (Evans, 1951: 129).
155 x 55 mm.
Loaned by Dr. David Wilkinson, St. Bartholomew's Hospital.

235. GOLDMAN'S VINESTHENE DRIP
1940–60 *A.C. KING/LONDON*
A 25cc bottle for Vinesthene in a stainless steel jacket with window, the neck connected to control tap and drip, terminating in a T-junction tube, for connection to a Boyle's machine as a supplement to nitrous oxide anaesthesia (to achieve greater relaxation) (Minnitt and Gillies, 1945: 193).
170 x 85 x 45 mm.
Loaned by Dr. David Wilkinson, St. Bartholomew's Hospital.

236. GOLDMAN'S VINESTHENE INHALER
1940–60 *A.C. KING/LONDON*
A combined stopcock and spongebox for connection to a facepiece and 1 gallon rebreathing bag. The stopcock has three positions; fill, off and on.
The Goldman inhaler was designed for use in dental extractions lasting approximately 60 seconds. The contents of a 3cc ampoule of Vinesthene were placed, via the inlet funnel, on the sponge, the inlet valve closed and the outlet valve opened ready for use. In c. 1938 it cost £3.50 (Minnitt and Gillies, 1945: 192).
125 x 70 x 55 mm.
Loaned by Dr. David Wilkinson, St. Bartholomew's Hospital.

237. OXFORD VINESTHENE INHALER
1940–60 *A.C. KING*
A modification of the Goldman inhaler (above), the additional features being a one-way inlet valve to admit air on inspiration if the bag was deflated, and a by-pass control to permit a gradually increased dose of anaesthetic (Minnitt and Gillies, 1945: 192–3).
130 x 65 x 120 mm.
Loaned by Dr. David Wilkinson, St. Bartholomew's Hospital.

238. VINESTHENE British Oxygen Company Ltd., *Anaesthetic apparatus*, c.1950, Trade Catalogue, p.68. 'The Oxford Vinesthene Inhaler'. No price stated.

239. FLUOTHANE (Halothane)
1960–80 *IMPERIAL CHEMICAL INDUSTRIES LIMITED.*
Supplied in a 50 ml brown glass bottle with screw cap. Investigated in the laboratory and clinically in 1956, halothane rapidly came to be considered "one of the most useful agents in the whole history of clinical anaestheisa" (Wylie and Churchill-Davidson, 1972: 329). It was potent, non-flammable and non-irritating.
100 x 31 x 31 mm.
Loaned by Dr. David Wilkinson, St. Bartholomew's Hospital.

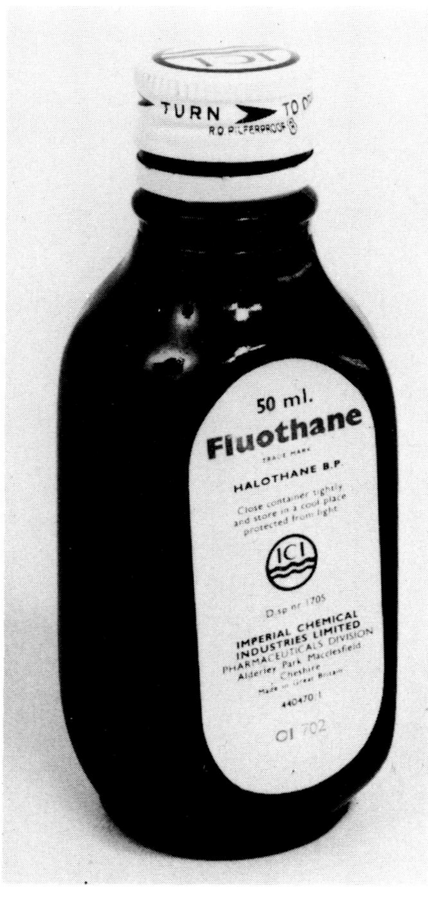

240. FLUOTHANE Photograph of an advertisement by Ayerst laboratories for Fluothane (Halothane) in *Anesthesiology*, 1962, *23*: 7–8.

241. PENTHRANE (Methoxyflurane)
1960–70 *Abbott Laboratories Ltd./Queenborough, Kent.*
Supplied in a 125 ml plastic-coated glass bottle. Methoxyflurane was one of a group of chemical compounds (known as fluorinated hydrocarbons) which were systematically investigated in the laboratory as potentially useful anaesthetic agents. Halothane (see above) belongs to the same group, which was identified on the basis of predicted effects of variations in molecular structure. Use of this agent declined rapidly in the 1970s, following reports that it damaged the kidneys.
112 x 47 mm.

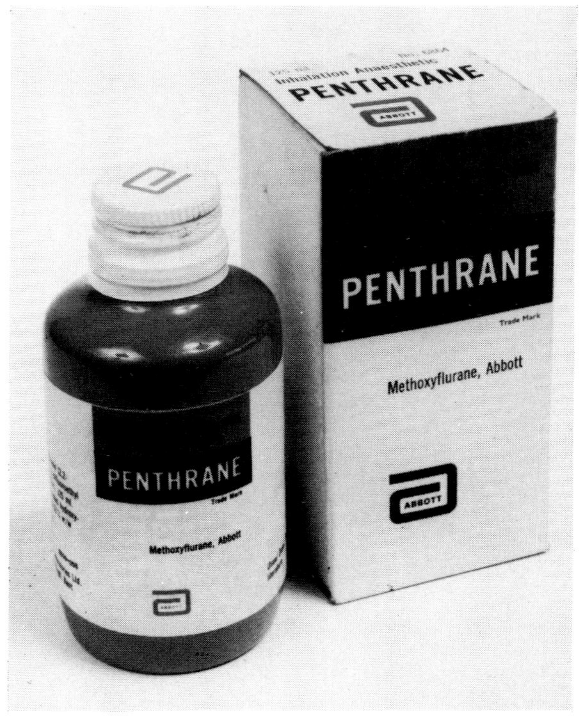

242. PENTHRANE Photograph of an advertisement for Penthrane in *Anesthesiology*, 1962, *23*: 50–1.

CASE 13: ANAESTHESIA AND THE CHLOROFORM QUESTION

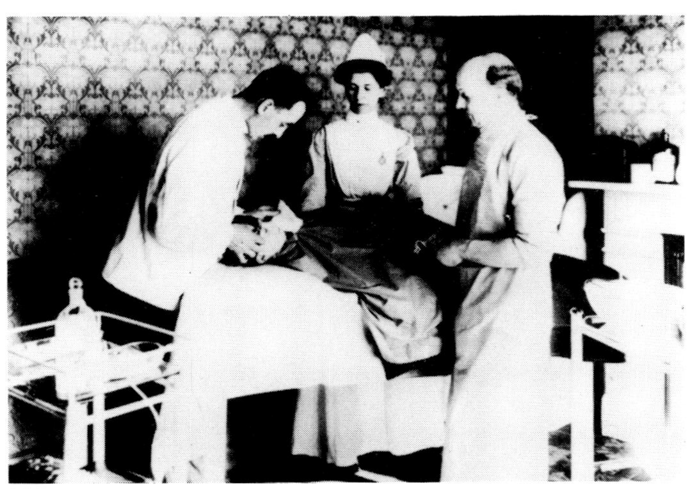

Item 244

The mode of action of anaesthetic agents has been an object of enquiry ever since the late 1840s. This enquiry has been pursued from two points of view. First, it has been undertaken by practising anaesthetists interested in the physiological basis of the clinical changes produced by inhalational agents. John Snow (1813–58), for example, undertook extensive investigations on ether and chloroform (see *Anaesthesia and the Victorians*). Second, anaesthetic agents have been investigated by professional physiologists. In this instance the drugs have usually been used as a means to pursue general physiological problems. Claude Bernard (1813–78), for example, worked extensively on curare and inhalational agents as part of his work on the neuromuscular system (Leake, 1971; Bernard, 1875).

Anaesthetic textbooks, of which the first comprehensive British work was Dudley Buxton's *Anaesthetics*, of 1888, have routinely included accounts of the physiological action of anaesthetic gases and vapours (Buxton, 1888). Perhaps no agent has been the focus of more physiological interest than chloroform. From the mid-1850s the safety, or otherwise, of chloroform was the subject of vigorous controversy. There were at least eight major British chloroform commissions and committees between 1864 and 1912 (Thomas, 1975: 61). The major features of these debates have been well described by Sykes, although there has been little investigation into the use of chloroform in routine practice (Sykes, 1960: 137–168). In the nineteenth century chloroform was widely used in Scotland, particularly in Edinburgh, where surgeons, on the authority of James Young Simpson (1811–70) and James Syme (1799–1870), considered chloroform very safe, and gave it by simple inhalation after pouring it on a folded towel (Buxton, 1888: 78). In general practice, according to one author, methods of giving chloroform were often quite slapdash: "Chloroform has generally been poured on freely from the original $\frac{1}{2}$lb. or 1lb. bottle, and no particular regard paid to the quantity used" (Luke, 1905: 52). In Scotland, anaesthetists were taught to watch the respiration while chloroform was administered, as an indication of possible complications. Anaesthetists in England, or at least in the major centres, often gave chloroform by using inhalers such as Snow's or Clover's, although they too used the Scottish method. Many London doctors insisted on the importance of monitoring the pulse as well as the respiration. Death, they claimed, could occur not only by respiratory failure, but also through cessation of the heart beat. Thus differences in the technique of chloroform administration in Scotland and England were accompanied by quite different claims about the drug's action and safety. These differences had become so pronounced by the late 1880s that a major enquiry was initiated into the physiological action of chloroform.

The man primarily responsible for this was a surgeon who had had great success in the use of chloroform, Surgeon – Major Edward Lawrie (1846–1915), Principal of the Hyderabad Medical School, and champion of the Scottish view (*BMJ*: 1889). In 1888 Lawrie enlisted the support of the Nizam of Hyderabad to finance a commission to investigate the action of chloroform. In 1889, before the Commission had published its findings, Lawrie announced that it had discovered that, after experiments on 128 dogs, death occurred by cessation of respiration and not by stoppage of the heartbeat. The *BMJ* reported that Lawrie "had no doubt deaths would go on occurring until the London Schools ... ignored the heart in chloroform administration" (*BMJ*, 1889). The *BMJ* along

with the *Lancet*, in this instance the voices of London medicine, did not concur. The Nizam offered
to finance a second enquiry under the supervision of a distinguished authority chosen by the British
profession. Thomas Lauder Brunton (1844–1916), physician and physiologist, was duly dispatched
to Hyderabad where he supervised the work of the Second Commission which reported, in 1890,
in the same manner as the first. London anaesthetists remained unconvinced however. In the
second edition of his work in 1892, Buxton reported the Commissions' findings, but he maintained
that chloroform could kill by "interfering with the heart's action" (Buxton, 1892: 100). London
anaesthetists continued to monitor the pulse, and physiologists, notably Leonard Hill (1866–1952),
offered experimental evidence to support their clinical claims and suspicions of dropper bottles,
masks and the open method (but see Hewitt 1901: 325).

In 1901 the British Medical Association set up a special Chloroform Committee under the chair-
manship of Augustus Desiré Waller (1856–1922) to inquire into the question. It reported in 1910.
The Committee recommended that chloroform should not be administered in concentrations higher
than two percent. To achieve this level a number of devices had already been contrived, notably by
Waller himself, Vernon Harcourt (1834–1919) and A. Goodman Levy (1866–1954). By the 1930s the
Scottish view was moribund and it was generally agreed that the heart could be primarily affected
by chloroform. This consensus, however, had little effect in practice as chloroform continued to be
given on masks. Neither Shipway's apparatus nor Boyle's apparatus, both of which could be used
to give chloroform, had any mechanism for controlling the amount (see *Anaesthesia and Technical
Solutions*). The end of the employment of chloroform came, not because of the results of physiological enquiry, but because of the introduction of new agents such as Halothane (see *Anaesthesia
and Industry: Two*).

CLAUDE BERNARD

243. RESEARCH Claude Bernard, *Leçons sur les
anesthésiques et sur l'asphyxie*, Paris, J.B. Baillière
et Fils, 1875. With the signature of Thomas Lauder
Brunton on the title-page.

HYDERABAD

244. PHOTOGRAPH showing the administration of
an inhalational anaesthetic, almost certainly chloroform, by the open method. The Wandsworth Medical
Centre, London, c. 1911. (Copyright Greater London
Photographic Library 80/0339)

245. INHALER *Description of the Hyderabad Chloroform Inhaler, or open-ended cone, with Krohne
Sesemann's Patent Respiration indicator with direc-
tions for use as given by Surgeon-Major Edward
Lawrie*. Pamphlet, produced by the instrument makers, Krohne and Sesemann, London, to sell the Hyderabad inhaler, c. 1891. (Loaned by The Pharmaceutical Society)

246. CHLOROFORM Edward Lawrie, *Chloroform:
a manual for students and practitioners*, London, J.
& A. Churchill, 1901. Dedicated to His Highness the
Nizam of Hyderabad.

247. COMMISSION C.H. Leaf, J.A. Kelly and A.
Chamarette, *Experiments with chloroform and ether
conducted at Hyderabad (Deccan)*, Bombay. Printed
at the "Times of India" Steam Press, 1892. Annotated by an unknown hand, possibly one of the authors. This is the Report of the First Chloroform
Commission, which was not published until 1892,
three years after the Report of the Second Commission.

248. COMMISSION *The Lancet and the Hyderabad
Commissions on chloroform*, London, Offices of The
Lancet, [1893]. Containing the Reports of the two Hyderabad Commissions of 1889 and 1890 (both slightly
ammended) and *The Lancet* Commission of 1893.
Showing 'General view of the apparatus employed'
by the Second Commission p. 72.

DOSIMETRIC METHODS

249. ANAESTHETIC CHLOROFORM
1959 *PHILIP HARRIS & Co. (1913) Ltd./
PHARMACEUTICAL SPECIALISTS,/
BIRMINGHAM.*
Supplied in a ridged brown glass poison bottle with
ground glass stopper and printed paper label, dated
13 June 1959, priced 10d.
200 x 68 mm. 1987–145

250. A.D. WALLER'S CHLOROFORM BALANCE
1884–1903 *BAIRD AND TATLOCK/*
(LONDON) LTD.
A brass laboratory balance with a glass bulb marked
'560cc' suspended from one arm, the case adapted
so as to be filled with chloroform vapour by an electric air pump and chloroform bottles (now missing)
mounted to the frame. A counter-weight was used
such that the glass bulb rose with the increasing den-
sity of the mixed gases, the percentage of chloroform
being read from the handwritten scale, '0–1–2–3'.
A.D. Waller (1856–1922) used the balance to supply,
via an outlet tube, a known percentage of chloroform
in air, largely in work on laboratory animals. The
balance was "hardly applicable for everyday surgical use" (*BMJ*, 1910: 67). This example was owned
by him during his years as Lecturer in Physiology at
St. Mary's Hospital, London (1884–1903) (for his account of the balance, see Waller, 1910: 109).
550 x 470 x 270 mm.   1984–1668/2

251. DUBOIS ANAESTHETIZING MACHINE
c. 1900 *Mathieu, 113 Bd. St. Germain Paris.*
A metal drum containing a vaporizing chamber into
which a measured amount of chloroform is driven by
a piston at the same time as a measured volume of
air is drawn in by a pump, if the handle is turned
at a regular rate. The vapour reached the patient by
a flexible tube and valveless facemask (missing from
this example) or the oral and nasal tubes provided. A
spirit lamp heats a metal plate to warm the vaporizing chamber by conduction. The whole apparatus is
cased in a fitted, felt-lined, wooden box. Dubois' machine was advertised by the makers in their catalogue
of c. 1910 (Mathieu, c. 1910: 63).
The machine was devised by a physiologist, Raphaël
Dubois (1849–1929), who, with an engineer, worked
with Paul Bert (1833–86) during 1884–5 at the
Hôpital Saint-Louis, Paris.   A.D. Waller drew on

Bert's work and owned this example of Dubois' machine, which bears a serial no. 42 (for a detailed introduction to Bert's work on anaesthetics, and the use
of this machine, see Duncum, 1947: 356–74).
case 480 x 310 x 310 mm.   1984–1668/3

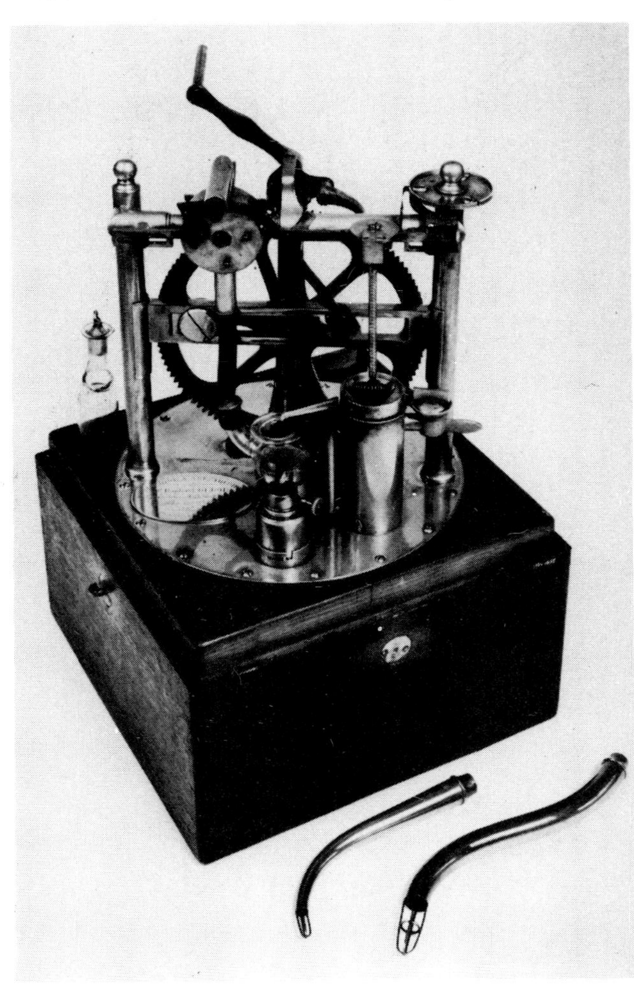

252. VERNON HARCOURT Inhaler
1903 *Griffin. London.*
This example is fully described elsewhere (Thomas,
1975: 86–9). A.G. Vernon Harcourt (1834–1919) was
Reader in Chemistry at Christ Church, Oxford and
was closely involved with the work of the Chloroform
Committee of 1901. His inhaler, designed to deliver
known percentages of chloroform up to two percent,
appeared in 1903 (*Lancet*, 1903). This example is
provided with a stand and heating candle for the
chloroform bottle. Others could be hung round the
administrator's neck (see Buxton, 1914: pl.v.). Unlike Levy's inhaler (see *Anaesthesia and the Cardiologist*), Vernon Harcourt's did appear frequently in
textbooks and manufacturers' catalogues. In 1906 it
cost five guineas, a 'non percentage' inhaler for chloroform, such as Junker's, costing £1–6s (Down, 1906:
1071,4).
386 x 240 x 228 mm.
Loaned by The Charles King Collection, Association
of Anaesthetists of Great Britain and Ireland.

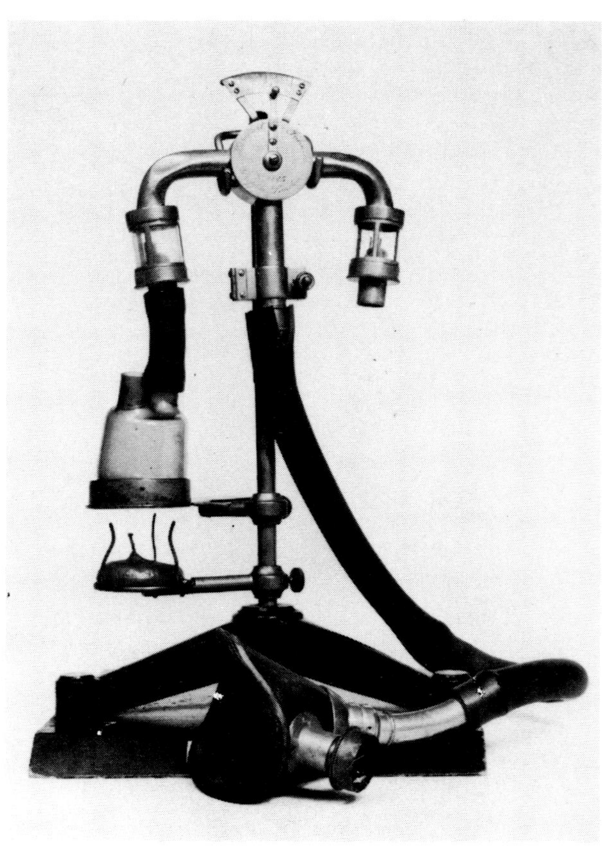

255. COMMISSION British Medical Association, *Report of the Special Chloroform Committee*, London, British Medical Association, 1911. Originally published as a supplement to the *BMJ*, 1910, *ii*: 47–72. Dudley Buxton, Honorary Secretary of the Committee, wrote in the foreword that chloroform was still used in much the same way that it had been by Simpson and Snow and that the "death rate has increased year by year". The *Report* came out strongly in favour of dosimetric methods of administration and against the open method.

253. PHOTOGRAPH of an operation at St. Bartholomew's Hospital, c. 1910. The anaesthetist, Charles Hadfield (1875–1965), is using a Vernon Harcourt apparatus. Hadfield was also a champion of open ether (*Lancet*, 1965). (From an original in the Illustrations Department, St. Bartholomew's Hospital)

254. PHOTOGRAPH of 'The New Operating Theatre', Great Northern Central Hospital, London. The anaesthetist seems to be using a Vernon Harcourt Apparatus.

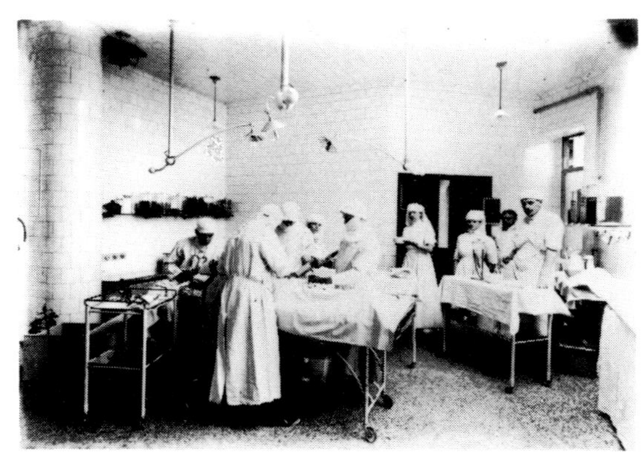

CASE 14: ANAESTHESIA AND THE CARDIOLOGIST

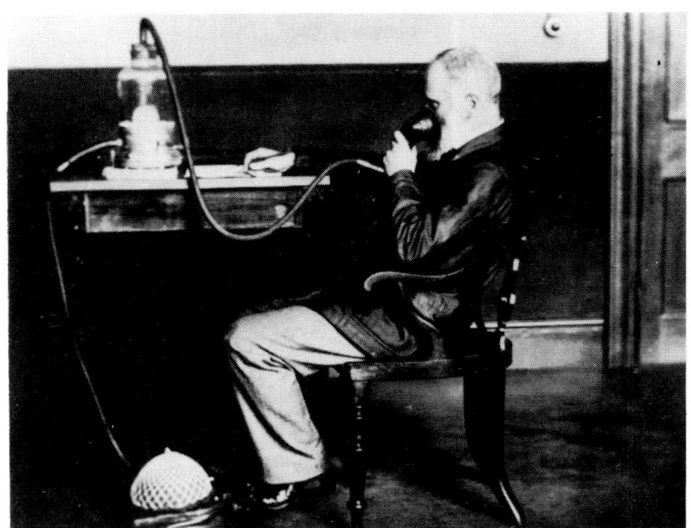

One of the photographs from Item 256

Until the recent disappearance of chloroform from the anaesthetic arsenal, the question of its action (if any) on the heart was vigorously debated in the medical literature. The reasons for these disputes lie as much in medicine generally as they do in the history of anaesthetics. One of the reasons why so much work was done on the action of chloroform on the heart was the emergence of cardiology as a specialty in the early twentieth century. At that time a 'new cardiology', as its practitioners called it, was created by employing new concepts, techniques and technologies. Using instruments derived from experimental physiology, such as the polygraph and the electrocardiograph, a few men reshaped the concept of heart disease to mean functional disorder rather than structural change (Lawrence, 1985). It was in this period that most of the modern terminology used to describe physiological and pathological rhythms was created. The most famous of these new cardiologists were Sir Thomas Lewis (1881–1945) and Sir James Mackenzie (1853–1925). Alongside these eminent physicians, however, were numerous other practitioners of various sorts, not necessarily heart specialists but men interested in applying the new cardiology to familiar problems. The action of chloroform on the heart was one of these.

The investigation into the effect of chloroform on the heart, therefore, was as much a part of the remodelling of ideas about the heart's action as it was part of the history of anaesthetics. The men who were bringing about the revolution in cardiology were using chloroform to understand cardiac physiology, besides investigating the heart to understand how chloroform acted. Thus Walter Holbrook Gaskell (1847–1914) and J.A. MacWilliam (1858–1937) who had investigated the muscular origin of the heart beat and the nature of ventricular fibrillation also published on the action of chloroform on the heart.

Around 1900, "heart failure", "paralytic dilatation", and "syncope" were the terms employed by anaesthetists who held that chloroform killed by its action on the heart (Buxton, 1902: 122; Hewitt, 1901: 89). It is often implied that the much disputed mode of action of chloroform on the heart was settled by various experiments, performed on cats, by Alfred Goodman Levy (1866–1954) (e.g. Keys, 1945: 76; Sykes, 1961: 82). Levy's work, first published in 1911 and in a number of subsequent papers, was based on suggestions made by Arthur Cushny (1866–1926), professor of pharmacology at University College London (Levy, 1911). Both Cushny and Levy were important figures in the establishment of the new cardiology. Levy had worked with Thomas Lewis, and had also practised as an anaesthetist. Levy injected adrenaline into lightly chloroformed cats and produced a graphic record of a form of cardiac arrest similar to that produced when the cats' hearts stopped spontaneously during chloroform anaesthesia. This work is now designated 'classic', but it was far from being hailed as definitive for many years (see Hovell, 1972). A survey of anaesthetic texts for the forty years following Levy's work shows that controversy over chloroform's action did not abate. Nor did Levy's work seem to have any immediate impact on the use of adrenaline after chloroform (Thomas, 1975: 89). The most important result of all this cardiac work, which probably only marginally improved the safety of administration of chloroform, was to facilitate the establishment of the methods and the techniques of the new cardiology and to encourage research into new anaesthetic agents.

256. FOUR PHOTOGRAPHS of A.D. Waller at work in a laboratory, n.d. (From originals marked 'Central Photographic Department, University of Liverpool' in WMSM)

257. WALLER'S MODEL TRAIN used in making ECG recordings
1887-1903
Model train wagon and track used by A.D. Waller in his electrocardiographic work at St. Mary's Hospital, London. His early methods involved the use of a slowly-moving photographic plate to record the electrocardiograph (Waller, 1887). The model wagon was apparently used to carry such a plate at a uniform rate, controlled by the clockwork mechanism. The plate which accompanies this set has a photograph of an electrocardiographic trace pasted to it, on which is typed "Fig. 1. *J. Physiol.* 1887. *Vol 8* p. 229". The wagon may have been used by Waller in lecture demonstrations, at which he apparently excelled (Burch and DePasquale, 1964: 97–108).
500 x 100 x 300 mm. 1984–1668/5

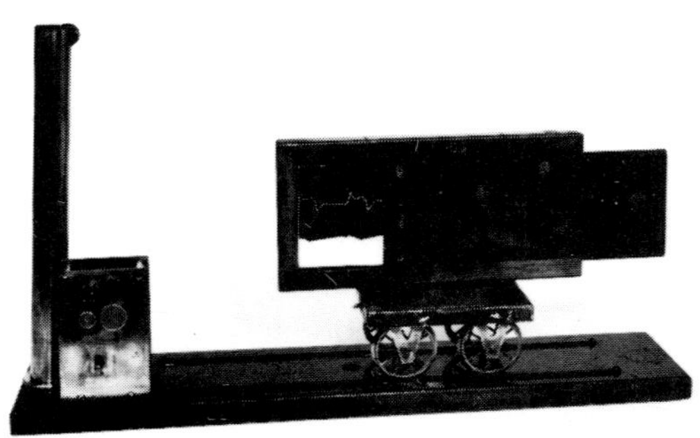

ELECTROCARDIOGRAPHY

258. CAMBRIDGE PORTABLE Electrocardiograph
c. 1940 *CAMBRIDGE INSTRUMENT Co LTD. ENGLAND.*
The recording apparatus, based on an Einthoven galvanometer, is enclosed in plastic and has an aluminium cover. It comprises a camera, a light source and film drums for producing the electrocardiographic trace from the movement of a string galvanometer. The model number of this example is C288771. It was an "all-mains" outfit apparently introduced by the Company in 1936, as an improvement on their first portable model of 1929 (Cambridge Instrument Co. Ltd., 1929; ibid.: 1936). It proved extremely popular.
The invention of the electrocardiograph permitted various interesting pieces of research work to be done on the anaesthetized patient. Once again, however, this was as much a part of cardiology as of anaesthetics (see e.g. Hill, 1932).
550 x 300 x 280 mm. 1979–203

259. PHOTOGRAPH of a physiology laboratory, University College London, 1925. (From an original in the possession of the Physiological Society)

260. PHOTOGRAPH of *The Illustrated London News*, October 30, 1909, p. 607 'Respiratory physiology experiments'. Showing experiments conducted under the supervision of Leonard Hill (1866–1952) at the London Hospital Medical School "to prove that oxygen is more sustaining than air".

261. CHLOROFORM A. Goodman Levy, 'Sudden death under light chloroform anaesthesia', *Journal of Physiology*, 1911, *42*: iii–vii.

262. A.G. LEVY'S REGULATING CHLOROFORM INHALER
1905–25 *MAYER & PHELPS.*
A drum-shaped, metal container holds a water jacket with thermometer, surrounding a chloroform vaporizing chamber. Movement of a pointer across a percentage scale (0.5-4, with corrections for temperature) alters the amount of air allowed to pass over the chloroform and hence the percentage mixture produced. A spherical mixing chamber above the drum has a permanently open air aperture. This was a special feature of Levy's design which ensured considerable dilution of the highly charged chloroform vapour (*Lancet*, 1904; Levy, 1905). An inspiratory valve, flexible tubing and facepiece with expiratory valve convey the mixture to the patient. The inhaler was designed to remedy faults Levy found in Vernon Harcourt's design (see *Anaesthesia and the Chloroform Question*) (Levy, 1922: 123). It was originally made by T. Hawksley, London. The maximum percentage of chloroform delivered was four percent.
535 x 360 x 213 mm. A625534

263. CHLOROFORM A. Goodman Levy, *Chloroform anaesthesia*, London, John Bale, Sons & Danielsson, Ltd., 1922, with a foreword by Arthur R. Cushny.

CASE 15: MONITORING IN ANAESTHESIA

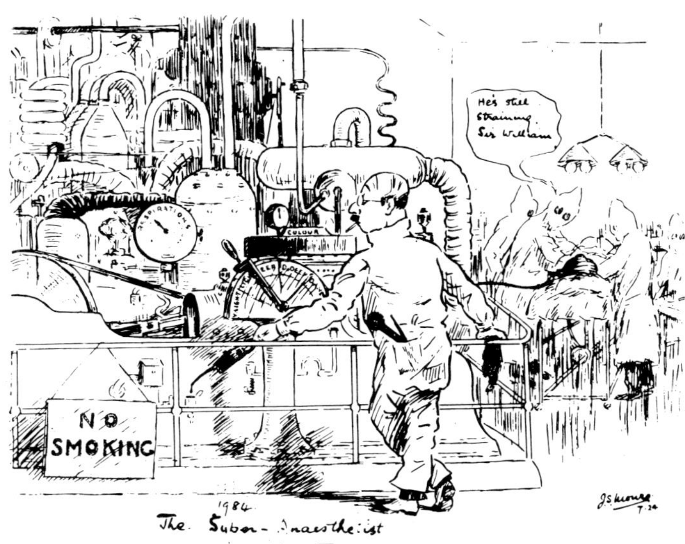

Item 265

Monitoring within anaesthesia is used here to mean several related things: the keeping of statistical records, the observation of a patient before, during and after an operation, and the monitoring of the rate of administration of anaesthetic agents. All these things have now become necessary requirements for normal anaesthetic practice. Monitoring and recording in standardized ways are crucial to modern medicine, yet their significance for understanding medical concepts and practice remains under-researched (Reiser, 1984). The same is true in anaesthesia. Stanley Sykes looked in some detail at the early chloroform statistics but this, apart from a few other exceptions, is about the extent of the historical enquiry into such areas (Sykes, 1961: 26–43). There are no good, detailed, empirical studies of how and why recording systems were conceived or made and for what purposes. Necessarily therefore there are no studies of how changes in monitoring practice have changed the ways in which anaesthetists have seen their role.

In the nineteenth century anaesthetists began to create rules to be observed when patients were examined before operation, and to indicate which anaesthetic agents were to be used in which circumstances; pure ether was contraindicated in arterial disease for instance (Buxton, 1888: 15). Rules such as these, however, give the historian no idea about actual practice. One author confessed that often there was no time to prepare the patient for operation (Probyn-Williams, 1901: 3). Victorian texts recommended that, during operations, the respiration be watched and the pulse felt. This latter was not an invariable rule, indeed, it was widely held, especially in Scotland, that it was positively contraindicated when giving chloroform, since the first signs of trouble were always indicated by respiratory change (Hewitt, 1901: 15) (see *Anaesthesia and the Chloroform Question*).

Nineteenth century anaesthetists had no obligation to make operation notes and it is likely that many of the details of anaesthetic practice in the past are irrecoverable. Joseph Clover (1825–82) did make notes after some operations. When he anaesthetised "H.M. The Emperor of the French" on December 26, 1872, he wrote:

> H.M. became insensible in three minutes without struggling or coughing. At the end of five minutes, slight stertor having been produced, Sir Henry Thompson commenced to explore the bladder. In a few minutes he recovered from the chloroform without sickness, depression or headache (Moorat, 1973: MS 1693).

Not only did anaesthetists rarely make operation notes, many did not keep a record of operations performed, and so data for the number of anaesthetics given and the incidence of complications or death are not easily discovered. Some anaesthetists, however, did keep figures and a few published them (see *Anaesthesia and the Victorians*).

In 1901 Frederic Hewitt (1857–1916) included detailed instructions for examining the patient in his *Anaesthetics and their administration*. There was, however, no section on recording or monitoring during operations. It is clear, however, that he assumed that the anaesthetist would watch the pulse, respiration, pallor, pupils and conjunctival and corneal reflexes (Hewitt, 1901).

In 1920, in America, the National Anaesthesia Research Society published a specimen record chart which it advocated should be used throughout the country in order to make uniform reporting possible. It included space for pre-operative and post-operative details with an area for the graphic recording of pulse, blood pressure and respiration. Sphygmomanometers were in use in this period but were far from common. In Britain there seems to have been far less inclination to record and standardize. Blomfield, in his textbook of anaesthetics of 1922, recommended preoperative X-ray and electrocardiographic examination if the anaesthetist was doubtful of the patient's ability to withstand anaesthesia. He also recommended the routine taking of the recumbent and erect blood pressure before operation. He noted that "By taking frequent readings of the blood pressure the anaesthetist is able to warn the surgeon ... that the patient is approaching a state of shock" (Blomfield, 1922: 327). This was written in such a way as to suggest that the taking of blood pressure was desirable rather than necessary, except when circulatory depression was evident from the pulse. Without an assistant, of course, it would have been very difficult for anaesthetists in the twenties to have taken the blood pressure. When Henry Souttar first operated on a patient with mitral stenosis at the London Hospital in 1925, the anaesthetist was a surgeon, and the surgical registrar took regular recordings of the systolic pressure (Ellis, 1975). Such attention was, probably, extremely unusual.

Things changed slowly over the next twenty years. In 1943, an anaethetist practising in Newcastle wrote "Most hospitals and surgical clinics today use an anaesthetic record or chart" (Ayre, 1943: 180). He also noted that some charts included "everything from the Basal Metabolic Rate to the anaesthetist's fee"(Ibid.). The chart he described contained space for a single, systolic, blood pressure reading. In America by this time a comprehensive, standardized punch card system was in use (Nosworthy, 1943). The reasons for this were as much political as clinical, being related to the accreditation system in use for American hospitals and the more general regulation of medical work in comparison to Britain. Monitoring of the patient, of course, changed profoundly with the electronics revolution in medicine in the 1960s and 70s. There was, however, no simple cause and effect relationship in this transformation; it was also a part of the changing and expanding role of the anaesthetist in medical practice. The anaesthetist to some extent ceased being a general practitioner or an itinerant carrying his own apparatus and became a specialist hospital employee using large, immobile apparatus installed in the hospital. Monitoring of women in labour and the move from home to hospital delivery illustrates nicely the complex change in social relations involving new monitoring practices (see *Anaesthesia and Women*).

BACK TO THE FUTURE

264. PHOTOGRAPH of a surgical operation at St. Bartholomew's Hospital, c. 1900. The anaesthetist is shown feeling the patient's temporal artery. He seems to be giving chloroform on a mask. (From an original in St. Bartholomew's Hospital, Illustrations Department)

265. PHOTOGRAPH of a cartoon depicting 'The Super-Anaesthetist 1984', by J.S. Monro, July, 1924. Location of original unknown. It depicts the anaesthetist of 1984 observing his complicated machinery, while the surgeon remarks of the patient, "He's still straining, Sir William".

266. PHOTOGRAPH Photograph of an anaesthetist and monitoring equipment during an operation in St. Bartholomew's Hospital, 1981. (From an original in St. Bartholomew's Hospital, Illustrations Department)

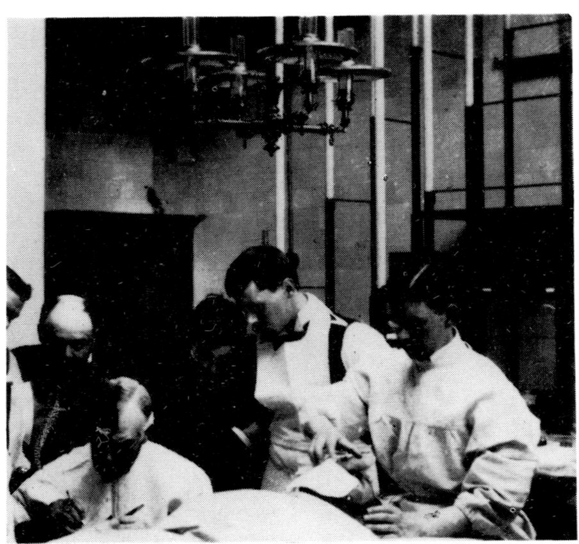

Item 264

267. 'DRY' FLOWMETERS
c.1935 *COXETER'S FLOWMETER*
Glass cylinder containing three glass tubes of uniform bore, with a series of holes drilled at intervals throughout their length, and connector to gas supply at base. Close fitting bobbins are forced up the calibrated tubes to a degree proportional to the flow of gas. Flowmeters of this type were introduced for use on anaesthetic machines between 1931–1933 (Watt, 1968: 107–8). They replaced the simple water sight-feed bottles through which anaesthetic gases were bubbled to provide an estimate of flow before being passed to the patient.
250 x 145 x 85 mm.
Loaned by Dr. David Wilkinson, St. Bartholomew's Hospital.

268. ROTAMETER FLOWMETERS
1961–75 *BOC. COXETER/KING/MEDICAL SECTION.*
An attachment for an anaesthetic machine comprising, within a metal housing, three tapered glass tubes, each calibrated to indicate the flow of the gas entering at the base (carbon dioxide, oxygen or nitrous oxide). A bobbin, cut with diagonal slits in its margin, spins in each tube, reaching a height proportional to the gas flow. In this example, the gases pass from the top of the housing through two Boyle's bottles for the vaporization of liquid anaesthetic agents. Rotameters of this type had been used in industry to measure gas and liquid flows and were adapted for anaesthetic use in 1937 – an innovation that has been the subject of a priority dispute (Watt, 1968: 111). The rotameter, more accurate than the Coxeter dry bobbin flowmeter (see above), became a standard fitting for anaesthetic machines from the late 1940s onwards.
420 x 160 x 210 mm. 1986–447

PHYSIOLOGICAL RECORDING

269. SHERRINGTON-STARLING KYMOGRAPH
c.1950 *C.F. PALMER (LONDON) LTD./63A EFFRA RD,/LONDON S.W.2.*
A revolving drum for smoked paper, mounted on a cast iron base with levelling screws and variable speed mount for a motorised belt-drive. A trace was produced on the smoked paper as the drum revolved, by means of a marker (missing from this example) which moved in response to, for example, the contraction of a muscle fibre to which it was indirectly connected.
The kymograph, devised by Karl Ludwig (1816–95) the Leipzig physiologist, was the fundamental recording instrument of experimental medicine (Hoff and Geddes, 1974). Modern monitoring equipment, which uses quite a different technology, employs the same principle: that the body's activities can be translated into a meaningful trace.
250 x 220 x 460 mm. 1979–714

270. WALLER'S GALVANOGRAPH
c. 1885
A light-tight metal box mounted on a wooden base, housing a revolving cylinder for light-sensitive (bromo-gelatine) paper. At the rear, a sliding panel allows access to the cylinder, and at the front a horizontal slit allows the deflection of a beam of light, reflected from the mirror of the accompanying Thompson's galvanometer, to mark the light-sensitive paper as the cylinder revolves (by clockwork). Using this type of apparatus, Waller obtained a record of the electric current flowing through muscle preparations, as part of his work on fatigue, carried out at St. Mary's Hospital, Paddington (Waller, 1885). This example differs slightly from that described by Waller in that the horizontal slit has no scale, but is covered by a glass capillary tube, clipped in place.
460 x 150 x 210 mm. 1984/168–12

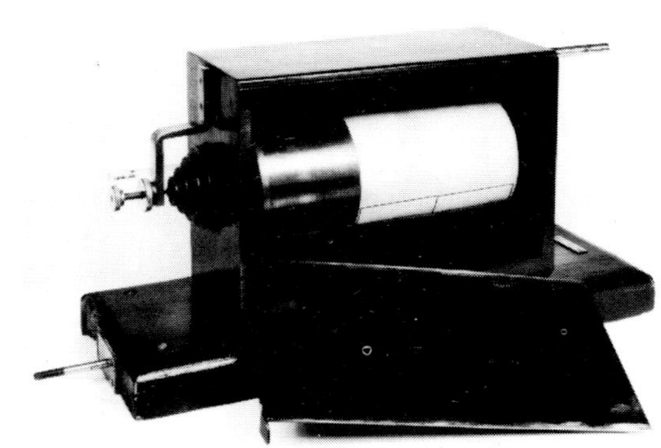

271. PHOTOGRAPH of an engraving of the recording apparatus used by Augustus Waller in his experiments on fatigue, published in 'Report on experiments and obsevations relating to the process of fatigue and recovery' *The British Medical Journal*, 1885, *ii*: 136. See the entry above.

272. MARTIN SPHYGMOMANOMETER
1900–20 *HAWKSLEY & SONS/357, OXFORD ST./ LONDON. W.*
Mercury and glass manometer tube, with engraved ivory scale, fitted, with leather and fabric arm-cuff, rubber tubing and hand bellows, into a cloth-covered wooden case. A metal mount supports the manometer in a vertical position when in use.
Sphygmomanometers, devised to study blood pressure within German physiological medicine of the late nineteenth century, remained specialized pieces of medical technology in Britain until the 1920s (Lawrence, 1979). Eventually, regular recording of the blood pressure became mandatory in anaesthetic practice.
case 391 x 125 x 68 mm. A600396

273. CAMPBELL-HALDANE APPARATUS
1960–75 *AIMER PRODUCTS LTD., 56–58
ROCHESTER PLACE/CAMDEN ROAD.
LONDON.*
A wooden carrying case with double doors and a central partition, to which is attached a glass gas burette within a water jacket. This is connected below to a mercury levelling bulb, and above to an absorption pipette containing potassium hydroxide. Two gas bags, for the collection of expired air from the patient, are stored in a rear compartment. Samples of air are injected into the gas burette and potassium hydroxide allowed to absorb the contained carbon dioxide, enabling its percentage in the sample to be estimated.

The British physiologist, J.S. Haldane (1860–1936) devised this equipment during studies on the composition of air in work places early this century (Haldane, 1920: 67–75). This modification was described in 1960 as more suitable for hospital use, where convenience and low cost were more important than a high level of accuracy (Campbell, 1960). Most Campbell-Haldane analysers were initially supplied to chest medicine units, as was this example. Anaesthetists began to make greater use of gas analysis techniques in the 1950s. Haldane-type apparatus such as this has been superseded by infra-red analysis (see below) and is now manufactured for sale in the Third World.
290 x 520 x 220 mm. 1985–2286/1

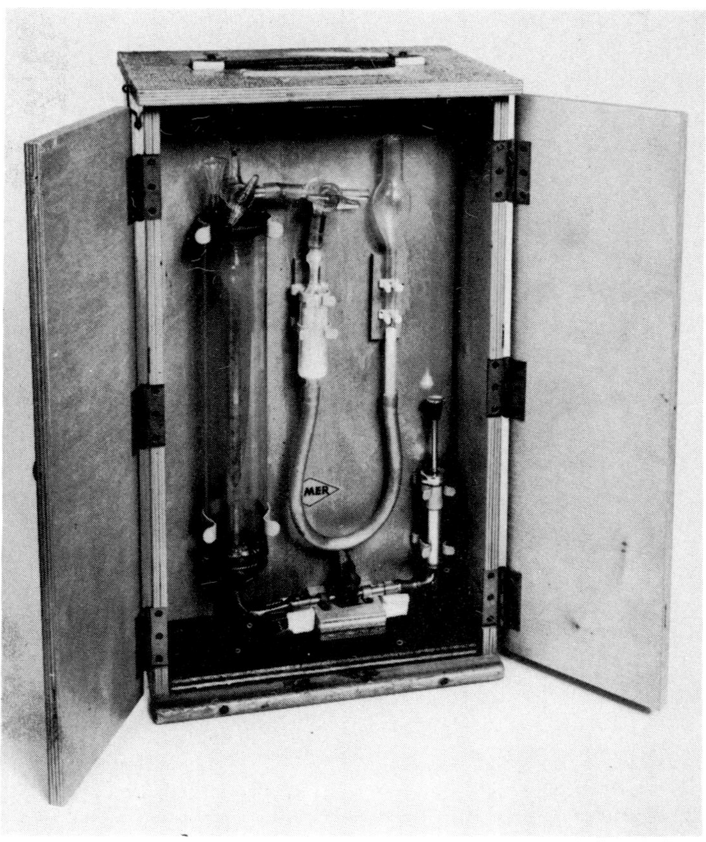

274. INFRA RED GAS ANALYSER
1955–75 *THE INFRA RED DEVELOPMENT CO.
LTD./WELWYN GARDEN CITY ENGLAND.*
An instrument used to determine the composition of a gas or vapour by comparing the wavelengths of infra-red radiation absorbed by a test sample and a sample of pure gas or vapour. The principle of the method was described in 1863 (Scurr and Feldman, 1976: 88). Anaesthetists began to use gas analysis for research purposes during the 1950s, when physical methods were superseding chemical ones (such as Haldane's, see above) (see e.g. Hill, 1960).

Infra red analysis is rapid, needing very small samples, and can therefore be used to monitor changing compositions of respiratory and anaesthetic gases.
470 x 230 x 520 mm. 1986–1078

RECORDS AND STANDARDS

275. 'ANAESTHESIA RECORD' a specimen record published by the National Anaesthesia Research Society in 1920.

276. RESEARCH F.H. McMechan (ed.), *Nitrous oxide-oxygen analgesia and anaesthesia in normal labour and operative obstetrics*, Columbus, Ohio, National Anaesthesia Research Society, 1920. Inscribed "To Mr. Henry Wellcome, in appreciation for many splendid services in behalf of the science and art of anaesthesia, with the compliments of The National Anaesthesia Research Society and the Editor". The Society was founded after a meeting of American anaesthetists in December 1919 (on McMechan, see Volpitto, 1982: 5–18).

277. CHARTS Philip Ayre, 'The anaesthetic record', *British Journal of Anaesthesia*, 1943, *18*: 180–4, showing the anaesthetic chart used at the Newcastle General Hospital.

278. BOYLE'S MACHINE
c. 1967 *THE BRITISH OXYGEN CO. LTD.*

A stainless steel framed trolley, with two formica shelves, to which the basic components of H.E.G. Boyle's (1875–1941) anaesthetic machine, originally described in 1917, are attached. These comprise gas cylinders – in this example, two of oxygen, one of nitrous oxide and one of cyclopropane, and bottles of liquid anaesthetic (in this example, ether and halothane) through which the gases are bubbled to effect vaporization. Other attachments include a row of rotameters (see *Monitoring in Anaesthesia*) to indicate rate of gas flow, an oxygen failure warning device, a sphygmomanometer to measure blood pressure and a soda-lime circle absorber to allow for closed circuit anaesthesia (see the essay in *Anaesthesia and Industry: One*).

Boyle's machine was first supplied in 1917 as a portable apparatus in a wooden crate. Its development as the basis of most subsequent British anaesthetic machines has been well documented (e.g. Watt, 1968).

1100 x 540 x 600 mm. 1986–1067

279. ENGSTRÖM RESPIRATOR Modell 150
1955–70 *MIVAB Electro-Medicinska Aktiebolaget/ Birger Jarlsgaten 66/ Stockholm.*

Within the housing of the ventilator an electric motor powers a piston which rhythmically drives air into the rigid plastic chamber mounted above, thus compressing the enclosed gas bag. From the gas bag, the air is forced into the patient's lungs via an endotracheal tube. The Engström was one of the artificial respirators designed in Europe in the years immediately following the Copenhagen poliomyelitis epidemic of 1952 (Engström, 1954). It became widely used for the new technique, introduced in the late 1950s, of temporarily paralyzing and artificially ventilating patients with actual or potential respiratory difficulties after surgery (Mushin *et al.*, 1969: 109–10). Specialized units were subsequently created in hospitals to provide the intensive monitoring and nursing care needed by these patients.

1460 x 1000 x 520 mm. 1987–225

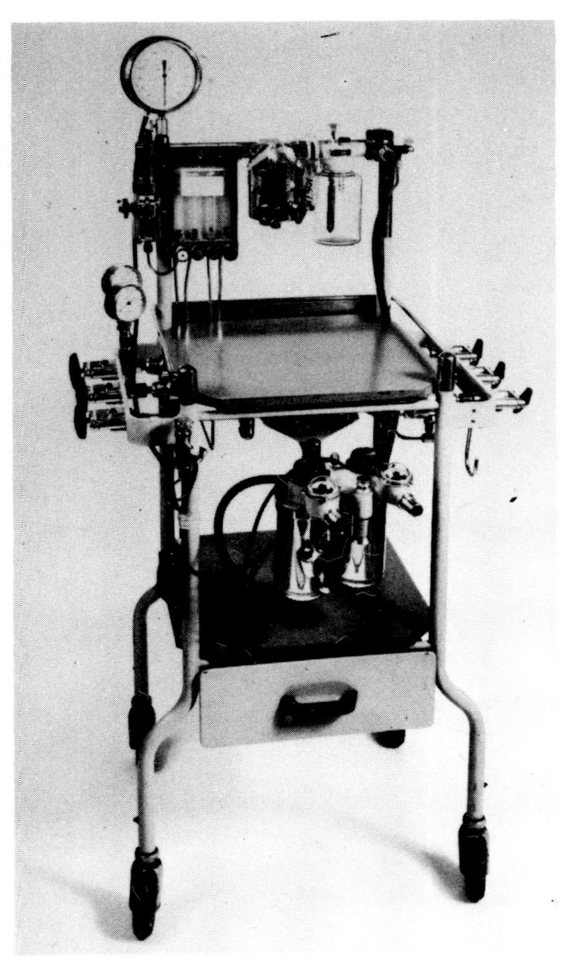

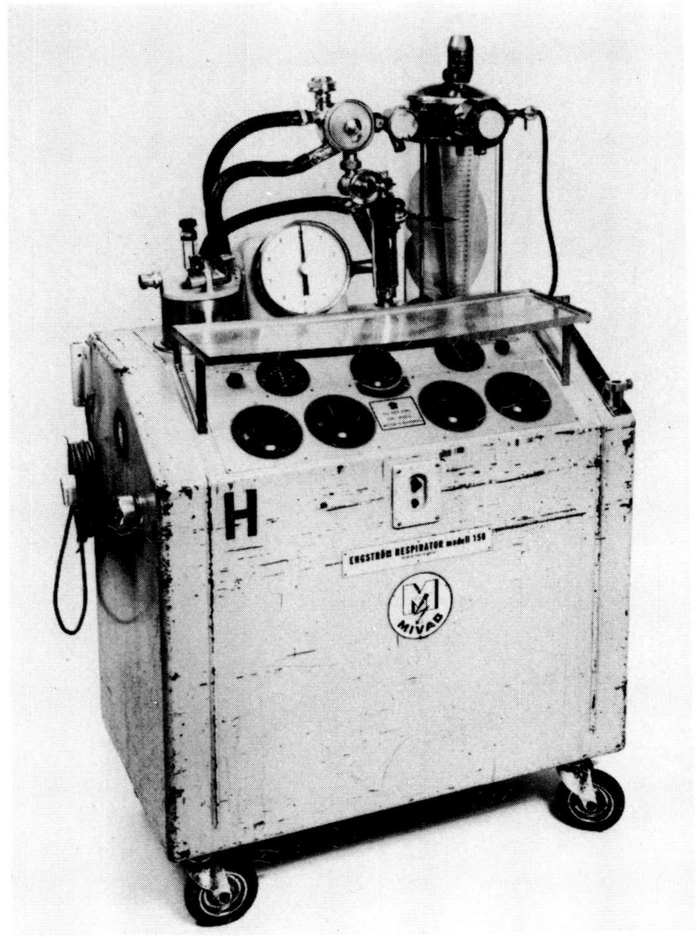

280. LUCY BALDWIN Analgesia Apparatus
1960–80 *BRITISH OXYGEN COMPANY
LIMITED. LONDON*
Oxygen and nitrous oxide cylinders are attached to
metal housing containing reducing valves and a sens-
ing diaphragm which allows a preselected mixture of
nitrous oxide and oxygen to flow when the patient
inhales from the facemask. In Britain, The Central
Midwives Board did not approve this machine for use
by a midwife (in the absence of a doctor) unless it was
'locked', such that the maximum concentration of nitrous oxide delivered was not more than fifty percent
(Wylie and Churchill-Davidson, 1972: 141–5). The
machine, developed in the late 1950s, was named after
Lady Baldwin (1859–1945), wife of the British Prime
Minister, who set up an anaesthetics fund to supply
nitrous oxide and air machines for labour wards in
1930 (Lewis, 1980: 129). A method of pre-mixing
oxygen with 50 or 60 percent nitrous oxide for com-
pression into cylinders (a technically difficult problem) was developed by The British Oxygen Company
from 1961, and this found widespread use in more
portable equipment for home and hospital confinements (the Entonox apparatus).
970 x 430 x 420 mm. 1984–1743

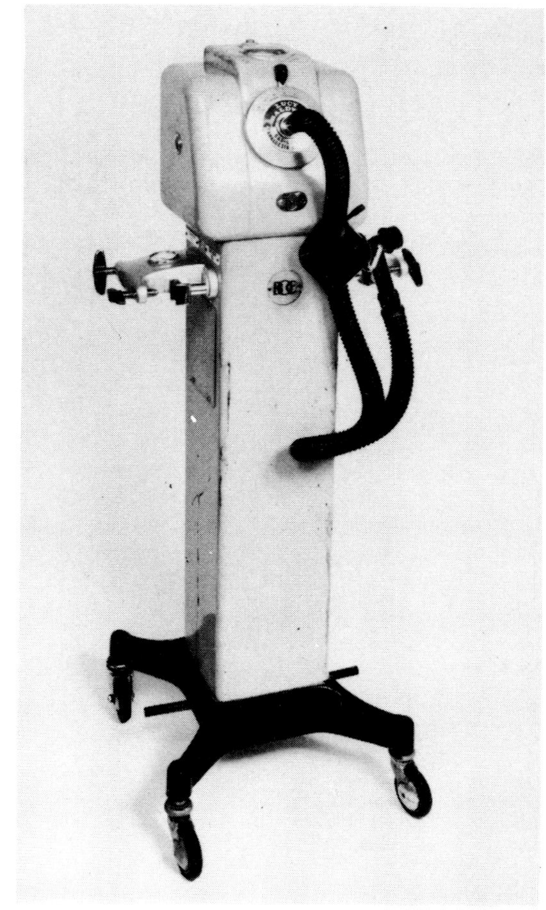

BIBLIOGRAPHY

Allen & Hanburys Ltd., *A catalogue of surgical instruments and medical appliances*, London, Allen and Hanburys, 1938.

Allen & Hanburys Ltd., *A reference list of surgical instruments and medical appliances* , London, Allen & Hanburys, 1930.

Allen, Carrol W., *Local and regional anesthesia*, Philadelphia and London, W.B. Saunders Company, 1918.

Anaesthesia, 'C. Langton Hewer', Obituary, 1986, *41:* 469–71.

Arnold and Sons, *A catalogue of surgical instruments*, London, Arnold and Sons, 1880.

Atkinson, R.S., and Boulton, T.B., 'Clover's portable regulating ether inhaler (1877)', *Anaesthesia*, 1977, *32*: 1033–6.

Ayre, Philip, 'The anaesthetic record', *British Journal of Anaesthesia*, 1943, *18*: 180–4.

Bader, C., 'The administration of chloroform and of other anaesthetics', *British Medical Journal*, 1870, *i*: 100.

Beaver, R.A., 'Pneumoflator for treatment of respiratory paralysis', *Lancet*, 1953, *i*: 977.

Bernard, Claude, *Leçons sur les anesthésiques et sur l'asphyxie*, Paris, J.B. Bailliére et Fils, 1875.

Blomfield, J., *Anaesthetics in practice and theory,* London, William Heinemann, 1922.

Bond, C. J., 'Ether-apparatus', *British Medical Journal*, 1884, *i*: 1157.

Boulton, T.B., 'The Department of Anaesthesia', *St. Bartholomew's Hospital Journal*, 1964, *68:* 303–6.

Boulton, T.B., 'Editorial', *Anaesthesia*, 1986, *41*: 469–71.

Boulton, T.B. (The Editor), 'Then and now', *Anaesthesia*, 1977, *32*: 898–903.

Braine, Charles Carter, 'A safety Junker inhaler', *British Medical Journal*, 1892, *i*: 1364.

British College of Obstetricians and Gynaecologists, *Investigation into the use of analgesics suitable for administration by midwives*, London, B.C.O.G., 1936.

British Journal of Anaesthesia, 'The nurse-anaesthetist controversy', 1941, *17*: 108–11.

British Medical Journal, 'Annotation', 1889, *i*: 429.

British Medical Journal, 'The annual museum', 1888, *ii*: 426.

British Medical Journal, 'Correspondence', 1868, *ii*: 44.

British Medical Journal, 'Dr. Richardson on the bichloride of methylene as a general anaesthetic', 1867, *ii*: 345.

British Medical Journal, 'ECT with curare', 1978, *i*: 48.

British Medical Journal, 'Ether and chloroform anaesthetic mixture', 1901, *i*: Epitome, 96.

British Medical Journal, 'An ether-inhaler', 1876, *i*: 567.

British Medical Journal, 'On anaesthesia by the rectal administration of the vapours of ether', 1885, *ii*: 659.

British Medical Journal, 'Report of the Special Chloroform Committee', 1910, *ii*: Supplement.

British Oxygen Co. Ltd., *Medical and clinical gases and gas equipment*, [c. 1937].

Brown, Laurence, *A catalogue of British historical medals, 1760–1960*, London, Seaby, 1980, vol. 1.

Burch, G.E., and DePasquale, N.P., *A history of electrocardiography*, Chicago, Year Book Medical Publishers Inc., 1964.

Burgess, Renate, *Portraits of doctors and scientists in the Wellcome Institute of the History of Medicine*, London, Wellcome Institute of the History of Medicine, 1973.

Burns, Stanley B., *Early medical photography in America (1839–1883)*, New York, The Burns Archive, 1983.

Buxton, D.W., *Anaesthetics. Their uses and administration*, London, H. K. Lewis, 1888.

Buxton, D.W., *Anaesthetics. Their uses and administration*, 2nd ed., London, H.K. Lewis, 1892.

Buxton, D.W., *Anaesthetics. Their uses and administration*, 3rd ed., London, H. K. Lewis, 1900.

Buxton, D.W., *Anaesthetics. Their uses and administration*, 4th ed., London, H.K. Lewis, 1907.

Buxton, D.W., *Anaesthetics. Their uses and administration*, 5th ed., London, H. K. Lewis, 1914.

Cambridge Instrument Company, Ltd., *Cambridge portable electro-cardiograph*, List no. 980, July 1929.

Cambridge Instrument Company, Limited, *Cambridge portable electro-cardiograph*, Supplement to List no 980, August 1936.

Campbell, E.J.M., 'Simplification of Haldane's apparatus for measuring CO_2 concentration in respired gases in clinical practice', *British Medical Journal*, 1960, *i*: 457–8.

Cartwright, F.F., *The English pioneers of anaesthesia*, Bristol, John Wright & Sons Ltd., 1952.

Claye, Andrew M., *The evolution of obstetric analgesia*, London, Oxford University Press, 1939.

Clover, J.T., 'Portable regulating ether-inhaler', *British Medical Journal*, 1877, *i*: 69–70.

Coates, W.M., 'Observations on chloroform and its administration', *Lancet*, 1851, *i*: 375–6.

Comrie, John D., *History of Scottish medicine*, 2nd ed., London, The Wellcome Historical Medical Museum, 1932, 2 vols.

Cope, Sir Zachary (ed.), *Surgery. (History of the Second World War. United Kingdom Medical Services)*, London, H.M.S.O., 1953.

Crellin, J.K., and Scott, J.R., *Glass and British pharmacy 1600–1900*, London, Wellcome Institute of the History of Medicine, 1972.

Dennis, Frederic Shepard, *The history and development of surgery during the past century*, [Philadelphia, 1905]. [Repr. from, *American Medicine*, 1905, *9:* 139–46, 181–7, 227–34, 265–71.

Donnison, Jean, *Midwives and medical men*, London, Heinemann, 1977.

Down Bros., Ltd., *A catalogue of surgical instruments and appliances*, London, Down Bros., Ltd., 1906.

Down Bros., Ltd., *Catalogue of surgical instruments and appliances*, London, Down Bros., 1935.

Duncan, Flockhart & Co., *The History of Duncan, Flockhart & Co.*, Edinburgh, 1946.

Duncan, Flockhart & Co., *Medical catalogue*, Edinburgh, Duncan, Flockhart & Co., 1946.

Duncum, Barbara M., *The development of inhalation anaesthesia*, London, Oxford University Press for The Wellcome Historical Medical Museum, 1947.

Ellis, Richard H., 'The first trans-auricular mitral valvotomy', *Anaesthesia*, 1975, *30*: 374–90.

Ellis, Richard H., 'The introduction of ether anaesthesia to Great Britain', *Anaesthesia*, 1976, *31*: 766–77.

Ellis, Robert, 'Additional note on anaesthesia by mixed vapours', *Lancet*, 1866, *i*: 509–10.

Ellis, Robert, 'Compound anaesthetics in midwifery', *Lancet*, 1866, *i*: 708.

Ellis, Robert, 'On anaesthesia by mixed vapours', *Lancet*, 1866, *i*: 144–5.

Ellis, Robert, *On the safe abolition of pain in labour and surgical operations, by anaesthesia with mixed vapours*, London, Robert Hardwicke, 1866.

Engström, C.G., 'Treatment of severe cases of respiratory paralysis by the Engström Universal Respirator', *British Medical Journal*, 1954, *ii*: 666.

Epstein, H.G., and Macintosh, R.R., 'Analgesia inhaler for trichlorethylene', *British Medical Journal*, 1949, *ii*: 1092–4.

Epstein, H.G., Macintosh, R.R., and Mendelssohn, K., 'The Oxford vaporiser no. 1', *Lancet*, 1941, *ii*: 62–7.

Evans, Frankis T. (ed.), *Modern practice in anaesthesia*, 2nd impression, London, Butterworth & Co. Ltd., 1951.

Flagg, P.J., *The art of anaesthesia*, revised 5th ed., Philadelphia, J.B. Lippincott Company, 1932.

Freedman, A., 'Trichloroethylene – air analgesia in childbirth', *Lancet*, 1943, *ii*: 696–7.

Freeman, S.E., *Medals relating to medicine and allied sciences in the numismatic collection of the Johns Hopkins University*, Baltimore, The Evergreen House Foundation, 1964.

Fulton, John F., and Stanton, Madeline E., *The centennial of surgical anesthesia*, New York, Henry Schuman, 1946.

Galley, A.H., 'The debt of anaesthesia to pharmacy', *Ann. Roy. Coll. Surg. Engl.*, 1964, *34*: 77–97.

Galley, A.H., and King, A. Charles, 'Modifications of the Clover's ether inhaler', *Anaesthesia*, 1948, *3*: 147–53.

Gardner, H. Bellamy, *A manual of surgical anaesthesia*, 2nd ed., London, Baillière, Tindall & Cox, 1916.

Gray, Henry M.W., *Treatment of war wounds*, Oxford, Oxford Medical Publications, 1919.

Gray, T.C., and Halton, J., 'A milestone in anaesthesia? (d-Tubocurarine chloride)', *Proc. Roy. Soc. Med.*, 1946, *39*: 400–8.

Griffith, H.R., and Johnson, G.E., 'The use of curare in general anaesthesia', *Anesthesiology*, 1942, *3*: 418–20.

Gwathmey, J.T., *Anesthesia*, New York, D. Appleton and Company, 1914.

Gwathmey, J.T., 'The story of oil-ether colonic anesthesia', *Anesthesiology*, 1942, *3*: 171–5.

Haldane, J.S., *Methods of air analysis*, 3rd ed., London, Griffin, 1920.

Halford, F.J., 'A critique of intravenous anaesthesia in war surgery', *Anesthesiology*, 1943, *4*: 67–9.

Hamilton, D., 'The nineteenth century surgical revolution; antisepsis or better nutrition?', *Bull. Hist. Med.*, 1982, *56*: 30–40.

Harbord, R.P., 'The teaching of anaesthesia to medical students', *British Journal of Anaesthesia*, 1954, *26*: 64–79.

Hardy, S.L., *A practical inquiry on the vapour of chloroform as a local application*, Dublin, Thomas Deey, 1854.

Hargrove, R.L., 'Awareness under anaesthesia', *Journal of the Medical Defence Union*, 1987, *3 (1)*: 9–11.

Hewer, C. Langton, 'Anaesthetic rooms', *British Medical Journal*, 1955, *ii*: 257.

Hewer, C. Langton, 'Forty Years on', *Anaesthesia*, 1959, *14*: 311–30.

Hewer, C. Langton, 'Obituary', *The Times*, 1986, February 1: p. 10.

Hewer, C. Langton, 'Obituary', *Anaesthesia*, 1986, *41*: 469–71.

Hewer, C. Langton, *Recent advances in anaesthesia and analgesia*, London, J. & A. Churchill, 1932.

Hewer, C. Langton and Hadfield, C.F., 'Trichlorethylene as a general analgesic and anaesthetic', *Proc. Roy. Soc. Med.*, 1941, *35*: 463–8.

Hewitt, F.W., *Anaesthetics and their administration*, 2nd ed., London, Macmillan, 1901.

Hill, D.W., 'The application of gas chromatography to anaesthetic research', in R.P.W. Scott (ed.), *Gas chromatography*, London, Butterworths 1960, pp. 344–51.

Hill, I.G.W., 'Human heart in anaesthesia; electrocardiographic study', *Edin. Med. J.*, 1932, *39*: 533–53.

Hoff, Hebbel E., and Geddes L.A., 'A historical perspective on physiological monitoring: Sherrington's mammalian laboratory and its antecedents', *Cardiovasc. Res. Cent. Bull. (Baylor Univ.)*, 1974, *13*: 19–39.

Hovell, B.C., Masson, A.H.B. and Wilson, J., 'Alfred Goodman Levy (1866–1954): a biography', *British Journal of Anaesthesia*, 1972, *44*: 115–21.

Jackson, Chevalier, *Endoscopie (bronchoscopie, laryngoscopie, oesophago-scopie) et chirurgie du larynx*, Paris, Librarie Octave Doin, 1923.

Jackson, D., 'A new ether drop bottle', *Lancet*, 1913, *ii*: 1779.

Jacyna, L.S., 'John Goodsir and the making of cellular reality', *J. Hist. Biol.*, 1983, *16*: 75–99.

Junker, F.E., 'Description of a new apparatus for administering narcotic vapours', *Med. Times and Gaz.*, 1867, *ii*: 590.

Keynes, Geoffrey (ed)., *Blood Transfusion*, Bristol, John Wright & Sons Ltd., 1949.

Keys, Thomas E., *The history of surgical anesthesia*, New York, Schuman's, 1945.

Lancet, 'Charles Frederick Hadfield', Obituary, 1965, *i*: 1402.

Lancet, 'Discussion of chloroform anaesthesia', 1904, *ii*: 1496.

Lancet, 'Society of anaesthetists', 1903, *i*: 800–3.

Lawrence, C.J., 'Moderns and ancients, the "New Cardiology" in Britain 1880–1930', in W.F. Bynum, C. Lawrence, and V. Nutton (eds.), *The emergence of modern cardiology*, London, Wellcome Institute for the History of Medicine 1985, pp. 1–33.

Lawrence, Christopher, 'Physiological apparatus in the Wellcome Museum. 3. Early sphygmomanometers', *Medical History*, 1979, *23*: 474–8.

Lazorthes, G., and Campan, L., 'The evolution of anesthesiology in brain surgery', *Journal of the International College of Surgeons*, 1954, *22*: 557–69.

Leake, C.D., 'Claude Bernard and anesthesia', *Anesthesiology*, 1971, *35*: 112–3.

Leibbrand, W., 'Die Gebrüder Bumm', *Berl. Med.*, 1965, *16*: 51–7.

Levy, A.G., *Chloroform anaesthesia*, London, John Bale, Sons & Danielsson, Ltd., 1922.

Levy, A.G., 'A regulating chloroform inhaler', *Lancet*, 1905, *i*: 1413–5.

Levy, A.G., 'Sudden death under light chloroform anaesthesia', *J. Physiol.*, 1911, *42*: iii–vii.

Lewis, Jane, *The politics of motherhood*, London, Croom Helm, 1980.

Luke, Thomas D., *A guide to anaesthetics*, 2nd ed., Edinburgh, William Green & Sons, 1905.

MacPhail, Angus, 'A survey of shock-therapy', *Electronics Forum*, 1949, *14*: 27–41.

Macpherson, W.G. et al. (eds.), *History of the Great War*, London, H.M.S.O., 1922, vol. 1.

Marshall, G., 'The administration of anaesthetics at the front', *British Medical Journal*, 1917, *i*: 722–5.

Mathieu, *Arsenal chirurgical*, Paris, Mathieu, [c. 1910].

Mayer & Meltzer, *An illustrated catalogue of surgical instruments and appliances*, London, Mayer & Meltzer, [c. 1914].

Medical Times and Gazette, 'Chloroform inhaler of Dr. John Murray', 1868, *i*: 540.

Minnitt, R.J., *Gas and air analgesia*, 2nd ed., London, Baillière, Tindall and Cox, 1944.

Minnitt, R.J., 'The history and progress of gas and air analgesia for midwifery', *Proc. Roy. Soc. Med.*, 1943, *37*: 45–8.

Minnitt, R.J., 'A new technique for the self-administration of gas-air analgesia in labour', *Lancet*, 1934, *i*: 1278.

Minnitt, R.J., and Gillies, J., *Textbook of anaesthetics*, 6th ed., Edinburgh, Livingstone, 1945.

Moorat, S.A.J., *Catalogue of western manuscripts on medicine and science in the Wellcome Historical Medical Library. II MSS. written after 1650 A.D.*, London, The Wellcome Institute of the History of Medicine, 1973, 2 vols.

Mushin, W.W., et al., *Automatic ventilation of the lungs*, 2nd ed., Oxford, Blackwell, 1969.

Mushin, W.W., and Rendell-Baker, L., *The principles of thoracic anaesthesia past and present*, Oxford, Blackwell Scientific Publications, 1953.

Nosworthy, M.D., *The theory and practice of anaesthesia*, London, Hutchinson Scientific, 1935.

Nosworthy, Michael, 'A method of keeping anaesthetic records and assessing results', *British Journal of Anaesthesia*, 1943, *18*: 160–79.

The Nuffield Department of Anaesthetics, University of Oxford, *The Oxford vaporiser*, [1941?].

Oakley, Ann, *The captured womb*, Oxford, Basil Blackwell Publishers Ltd., 1984.

Ormsby, L., 'The advantages of ether as an anaesthetic: with a description of a new inhaler', *British Medical Journal*, 1877, *i*: 451–3.

Ostlere, G., *Trichlorethylene anaesthesia*, Edinburgh, E. & S. Livingstone, 1953.

Ouvry, J.P.A., 'Medical Gases in Hospitals', *Hospital Management*, Jan/Feb 1971: 33–5.

Page, G. Scott, *Recollections of a provincial dental surgeon*, Chester-Le-Street, Casdec Limited, 1984.

Pernick, Martin S., *A calculus of suffering*, New York, Columbia University Press, 1985.

Pharmaceutical Journal, 'Apparatus for the administration of the vapour of ether', 1846–7, *vi*: 421–5.

Pharmaceutical Journal, 'Chloroform inhaler', 1847–8, *vii*: 313.

Pharmaceutical Journal, 'The chloroform inhaler', 1847–8, *vii*: 394.

Pharmaceutical Journal, 'Dr. Hedley's ether inhaler', 1846–7, *vi*: 587.

Pharmaceutical Journal, 'Dr. Snow's chloroform inhaler', 1847–8, *vii*: 441.

Pharmaceutical Journal, 'Ether inhaler, of Dr. Hedley (Bedford)', 1847–8, *vii*: 14.

Pharmaceutical Journal, 'On the inhalation of the vapour of ether', 1846–7, *vi*: 350–9.

Pinch, Trevor J., and Bijker, Wiebe E., 'The social construction of facts and artefacts: or how the sociology of science and the sociology of technology might benefit each other', *Social Studies of Science*, 1984, *14*: 339–441.

Probyn-Williams, R.J., *A practical guide to the administration of anaesthetics*, London, Longmans, Green and Co., 1901.

Proskauer, C., 'The simultaneous discovery of rectal anesthesia by Marc Dupuy and Nikolai Ivanovich Pirgoff', *J. Hist. Med.*, 1947, *2*: 379–84.

Read, Grantly Dick, *Revelation of childbirth*, 2nd ed., London, William Heinmann Medical Books Ltd., 1943.

Reiser, S.J., 'Creating form out of mass; the development of the medical record', in Everett Mendelsohn (ed.), *Transformation and tradition in the sciences*, Cambridge, Cambridge University Press 1984, pp. 303–17.

Rendle, Richard, 'On the use of protoxide of nitrogen gas; and on a new mode of producing rapid anaesthesia with bichloride of methylene', *British Medical Journal*, 1869, ii: 412–3.

Richardson, Benjamin W., 'On a new and ready mode of producing local anaesthesia', *The Retrospect of Medicine*, 1866, *53*: 369–84.

Rion, Hanna, *Painless childbirth in twilight sleep*, London, T. Werner Laurie Ltd., [1915].

Roderick, Gordon, and Stephens, Michael (eds)., *Where did we go wrong? Industrial performace, education and the economy in Victorian Britain*, Lewes, Falmer Press, 1981.

Ross, Stuart J., and Fairlie, H.P., *Handbook of anaesthetics*, 4th ed., Edinburgh, E & S Livingstone, 1935.

Rowbotham, E.S., and Magill, I., 'Anaesthetics in the plastic surgery of the face and jaws', *Proc. Roy. Soc. Med.*, 1921, *14*: 17.

Royal College of Surgeons of England, 'Descriptive catalogue of surgical instruments in the museum of the Royal College of Surgeons of England, Part 19, Section "S", Anaesthetic Apparatus', Unpublished typescript, 1952.

Rupreht, J., et al., *Anaesthesia. Essays on its history*, Berlin, Springer-Verlag, 1985.

Sandelowski, Margarete, *Pain, pleasure, and American childbirth*, Westport, Conn., Greenwood Press, 1984.

Sansom, A.E., *Chloroform: its action and administration*, London, John Churchill and Sons, 1865.

Schaffer, Simon, 'Scientific discoveries and the end of natural philosophy', *Social Studies of Science*, 1985, *16*: 387–420.

Schubach, William, 'A select iconography of animal experiment', in Nicolaas Rupke (ed.), *Vivisection in historical perspective*, Beckenham, Croom Helm, 1987 (In press).

Scurr, C.F., 'Evolution and revolution in anaesthetic training', *Ann. Roy. Coll. Surg. Engl.*, 1971, *48*: 274–92.

Scurr, C.F., and Feldman, S., *Scientific foundations of anaesthesia*, 2nd ed., London, William Heinemann Medical Books Ltd., 1974.

Seward, E.H., and Bryce-Smith, R., *Inhalation analgesia in childbirth*, Oxford, Blackwell Scientific Publications, 1957.

Seward, E.H., 'Self-administered analgesia in labour', *Lancet*, 1949, ii: 781–3.

Shipway, F.E., 'A new apparatus for the intratracheal insufflation of ether', *Lancet*, 1916, *ii*: 236.

Shipway, Francis E., 'The advantages of warm anaesthetic vapours, and an apparatus for their adminstration', *Lancet*, 1916, *i*: 70– 4.

Silk, J.F.W., *Modern anaesthetics*, 2nd ed., London, Edward Arnold, 1920.

Skinner, T., 'Chloroform administration', *British Medical Journal*, 1871, *i*: 490.

Smith, Protheroe, 'On the use of chloroform in midwifery practice', *Lancet*, 1847, *ii*: 572–4.

Smith, Truman, *Anaesthesia! The greatest discovery of the age! Who is entitled to the credit of it?*, New York, [1859?].

Smith, W.D.A., 'A history of nitrous oxide and oxygen anaesthesia. Part iv B. Further light on Hickman and his times', *British Journal of Anaesthesia*, 1970, *42*: 445–58.

Smith, W.D.A., *Under the influence. A history of nitrous oxide and oxygen anaesthesia*, London, Macmillan, 1982.

Snow, J., *On chloroform and other anaesthetics: their action and administration*, London, John Churchill, 1858.

Snow, J., 'On the inhalation of chloroform and ether', *Lancet*, 1848, *i*: 177–180.

Squire, William, 'On the introduction of ether inhalation as an anaesthetic in London', *Lancet*, 1888, *ii*: 1220–1.

Stephen, C.R., and Little, D.M., *Halothane (Fluothane)*, Baltimore, The Williams & Wilkins Company, 1961.

Sykes, W. Stanley, *Essays on the first hundred years of anaesthesia*, Edinburgh, E. & S. Livingstone Ltd., 1960, vol. 1.

Sykes, W. Stanley, *Essays on the first hundred years of anaesthesia*, Edinburgh, E. & S. Livingstone Ltd., 1961, vol. 2.

Sykes, W. Stanley, *Essays on the first hundred years of anaesthesia. Edited by Richard H. Ellis*, Edinburgh, Churchill Livingstone Ltd., 1982, vol. 3.

Sykes, W. Stanley, 'Letter to the Editor', *British Journal of Anaesthesia*, 1941, *17*: 126.

Syme, James, 'Excision of the tongue', *Lancet*, 1865, *i*: 115.

Taylor, F.L., 'Crawford Williamson Long', *Annals of Medical History*, 1925, *7*: 267–96, 394–424.

Thatcher, Virginia S., *History of anesthesia with emphasis on the nurse specialist*, Philadelphia, J.B. Lippincott Company, 1953.

Thomas, K. Bryn, 'The A. Charles King collection of early anaesthetic apparatus', *Anaesthesia*, 1970, *25*: 548–64.

Thomas, K. Bryn, *The development of anaesthetic apparatus*, Oxford, Association of Anaesthetists, 1975.

Thompson, W.E., 'The collection of anaesthetic apparatus in the museum of the Royal College of Surgeons of England', *Ann. Roy. Coll. Surg. Engl.*, 1962, *31*: 269–76.

The Times, 'Dr. C. Langton Hewer', Obituary, February 1, 1986.

Tracy, M., and Boyd, M., *Painless childbirth*, London, William Heinemann, 1917.

Traer, J.R., 'Surgical, medical and obstetrical instruments in the International Exhibition of 1862', *Med. Times. and Gaz.*, 1862, *ii*: 148–9.

Volpitto, Perry P., and Vandam, Leroy D., *The genesis of contemporary American anesthesiology*, Springfield, Illinois, Charles C. Thomas, 1982.

Waller, A.D., 'A demonstration on man of electromotive changes accompanying the heart's beat', *J. Physiol*, 1887, *8*: 229–34.

Waller, A.D., *Physiology, the servant of medicine*, London, 1910.

Waller, A.D., 'Report on experiments and observations relating to the process of fatigue and recovery', *British Medical Journal*, 1885, *ii*: 135–48.

Ward, C.S., *Anaesthetic equipment*, London, Baillière, Tindall, 1975.

Watt, O.M., 'The evolution of the Boyle apparatus 1917–67', *Anaesthesia*, 1968, *23*: 103–19.

Wells, Spencer, 'A note on methylene and other anaesthetics', *British Medical Journal*, 1888, *ii*: 1211.

Wylie, W.D., and Churchill-Davidson, H.C., *A practice of anaesthesia*, 3rd ed., London, Lloyd-Luke, 1972.

Youngson, A.J., *The scientific revolution in Victorian Medicine*, London, Croom Helm, 1979.

FILM

The Great Moment, 1944, Paramount, see *Haliwell's film guide* 2nd ed., London, Paladin, 1982, p. 435.